MEDICAL SCHOOL INTERVIEWS

A practical guide to help you get that place at Medical School

Over 150 questions analysed Includes Multiple Mini Interviews (MMI)

2nd Edition

Author
Olivier Picard
BSc (Hons) MSc
Communication Consultant
Managing Director of ISC Medical

Contributor
George Lee
MA (Cantab) MB BChir (Cantab) MRCS(Ed) FRCS(Urol) FEBU
Consultant Surgeon

Published by:
ISC Medical, 97 Judd Street, London WC1H 9JG

Contact details:
Email: enquiries@iscmedical.co.uk
Web: www.iscmedical.co.uk
Tel: 0845 226 9487

This edition:
ISBN13: 978-1-905812-05-9. First printed: July 2013
A catalogue record for this book is available from the British Library.

Previous edition:
First edition printed 2006-2012 under ISBN13: 978-1-905812-04-3

Printed in the United Kingdom by:
Purbrooks, Gresham Way, Wimbledon, London SW19 8ED

Contents

Preface

Over the years, medical school interviews have become both more complex and more competitive. The introduction of multiple mini interviews (MMI) in some medical schools has caused some concerns amongst candidates and the process is not helped by the fact that different medical schools use different criteria to recruit, which leads to confusion amongst applicants in relation to the amount and type of preparation they should do.

Know yourself and be personal

Before you can convince a handful of strangers that you are the candidate they are looking for, it makes sense to convince yourself. An interview is not so much about making bold claims such as "I have all the attributes required to study Medicine" as it is about proving it through facts. In truth, most candidates have never thought in any depth about what they have to offer and they consequently come unstuck when asked for evidence to support their claims.

One student once asked me how she should answer the question "Why do you want to study Medicine?" I asked her what had motivated her to apply in the first place, to which she replied that she had no idea and just thought Medicine would be "interesting". All she wanted was a good model answer when, in truth, if there was ever a model answer, it would by its very nature be self-defeating as many candidates would come up with the same one and what could have been a good answer would simply become a "rehearsed" or clichéd answer. In truth there are many good answers and, most importantly, good answers are always those which are personal.

Without taking the time to understand her own true motivations for Medicine, that student could never deliver a good answer if that answer was simply served to her on a plate; instead she first needed to take the time to reflect on her own situation in order to develop a good answer. An interview is about <u>your</u> personal story, <u>your</u> experience, <u>your</u> strengths and weaknesses, <u>your</u> opinions; it is not about regurgitating a ready-made answer. Throughout this book I will show you how you can achieve this.

Focus on techniques

Preparing for an interview does not mean that you have to learn the answers to all possible questions; indeed there are far too many of them to make this a realistic goal. Regurgitating ready-made answers is also a recipe for sounding rehearsed. Instead, it is vital that you learn to understand and appreciate the skills and attributes that examiners are aiming to test with each question and that you acquire a range of approaches and techniques that you can apply to any question.

In this book I will describe several techniques that you can use to derive content and structure to a wide variety of questions. Use those sensibly to simplify your preparation and make your approach more systematic.

Balance preparation and practice

Essential though it may seem, you should resist the temptation to undergo mock interviews or practise answering questions in real-time conditions until you have a good understanding of the interview process, what it tests and the range of techniques that you need to answer any question thrown at you. Practising under pressure when you are not ready could indeed be counterproductive and induce a feeling of helplessness and panic that you could really do without. Before you can practise under pressure, we would therefore advise that you take your time to work through a wide range of questions at your own pace. Some questions may take you one minute to deal with whilst others may take much longer than that, but that initial time investment will pay off substantially both during your practice runs and on the day of the interview itself.

Good luck!

Olivier Picard

How to use this book

The reading material

In this book, we have given you everything you need to be aware of in relation to the history of Medicine, the history of the NHS, the current NHS and ethical principles. You do not need to know absolutely everything and you certainly should not aim to remember any of it by heart. However, your interviewers will expect you to have a basic understanding of all those issues; so you should at least read it attentively.

The formal interview questions

All interview questions contained in this book are real and recent interview questions asked at various medical school interviews around the UK. There are obviously many others that could be asked, but those in this book have been chosen because they offer a good representation of the type and range of questions which may come up. We suggest that you first read the book from cover to cover to get a feel for the techniques used to answer the various questions. Once you have done that, you can then take each section one at a time so that you can work on your technique, practise and refine your approach.

This book contains many examples of good and bad answers. Their purpose is to give you an appreciation of what sounds good and bad and how answers can be improved so that you can apply a similar thinking process to your own answers. There are many types of bad answers but there are also many types of good answers. The examples in this book should be taken as illustrations of the techniques discussed and not as a blanket template. Instead of trying to replicate the answers faithfully, try to use them to understand each of the principles outlined and to determine how you can then apply these principles to your own situation.

The practical MMI stations

This book will also show you how to handle the various practical MMI stations that you may encounter. You can prepare for many of them simply by getting an understanding of the exercises and the skills that they are testing, which this book should help you with. For some of the stations, such as role play, you may wish to grab a friend who can play the opposite person for practice purposes.

THE

SELECTION

PROCESS

1 Structure of the interview and the meaning of MMI

The structure of the interview varies greatly from one medical school to another. Some medical schools have one simple traditional interview panel whilst others adopt a more complex approach that includes several stations, called MMI.

The term MMI (multiple mini interviews) refers simply to the fact that the interview process is based on several stations. It does not give any indication as to the nature of those stations. For example, some medical schools may have three or four stations in which they ask only traditional interview questions; other schools may use a mix of traditional questions and more sophisticated tools such as group discussions or role play.

Therefore, if you are invited to an MMI-style interview, do not make the mistake of assuming that you will not be asked traditional interview questions. You will most likely be asked traditional questions in at least two of the MMI stations (usually there is at least one station testing your interest in Medicine, and one station testing your critical and lateral thinking as well as your ability to discuss ethical situations).

One major advantage of the MMI approach is that candidates are tested by different interviewers/assessors in different stations and, as such, your performance is totally separate from your performance in other stations. In other words, if you mess up on one question or task, the bad impression you may have given will not affect the marking of the other questions or tasks. In addition, candidates who are uncomfortable in formal interview situations may find some of the MMI stations more suited to their personality. On the other hand, it means that you spend little time with any one interviewer/assessor; consequently, you don't have much time to build a rapport.

You should determine as early as possible the structure that each medical school to which you have applied will be using (be aware that some medical schools change their system every year and you cannot simply rely on the experience of previous years' candidates – check each medical school's website and enquire with the admissions office if necessary). You will then know what to expect when you turn up on the day of your interview and will also be able to tailor your preparation.

You will find it reassuring that, although the structure of the assessment varies from one medical school to the next, the number of activities and questions that can be asked of you is fairly limited and, as such, the fact that you may face different stations does not necessarily mean that your preparation time will be increased that much.

For example, in some medical schools, ethical questions can be asked either as part of a normal interview, or in a separate station using an article sent to you by post or by email some time before the interview. If you know how to handle ethical questions, you will be able to handle any scenario regardless of the format in which it comes.

Overall, the types of stations that you can encounter at interviews fall into two different categories:

- **Formal interview stations** i.e. those designed as traditional, formal question & answer sessions; and

- **Practical interview stations** i.e. those that require the performance of a task, individually or in groups, orally or in writing.

1.1 Formal interview stations

Formal interview stations take the form of one or more interview panels during which you will be asked a set number of questions in an allotted amount of time. The total length of the interview varies typically between 10 and 20 minutes. So for example, a 15-minute interview could consist of one panel for 15 minutes, or three panels of 5 minutes each. Interview panels usually contain two to four interviewers who are mostly doctors. Some medical schools also include medical students, academics or even nurses on their panels.

When there are several panels, each one will ask questions of a different nature, e.g. in a three-panel interview, one panel may focus on motivational questions, one may focus on interpersonal skills and the third one may focus on ethics and current issues.

The following topics will be covered in one or several stations:

- **Motivation, work experience and choice of medical school**
  Covers questions asking for your reasons for studying Medicine, your reasons for studying in that medical school, and questions relating to your personal statement and the teaching methods used at that medical school (such as PBL).

- **Knowledge and interest in medical-related issues**
  Covers discussions around current issues and reforms in the healthcare system, the role of Medicine in society, the role of the media in influencing the behaviours of patients and medical professionals, the history of Medicine (e.g. what you would regard as the most important medical advancement in the past 50 or 100 years) and any topic in which you may have shown an interest during your readings or work experience.

- **Interpersonal skills and personality**
  Covers questions relating to your communication, team playing and leadership abilities, as well as your ability to demonstrate empathy, and deal with stress, criticism and conflict. You may be asked how you would react to certain sensitive situations, to describe your strengths and weaknesses, and generally why you would make a good doctor.

- **Lateral thinking and creativity**
  Covers questions seeking your opinion on a variety of topics ranging from whether doctors should be involved in the regulation of contact sports, to the pros and cons of paying for your own care, or even whether it was a good idea to send a man to the moon, or how many uses you can think of for a mobile phone charger.

- **Ethics and dilemmas**
  Covers discussions around ethical issues such as euthanasia and animal testing and debates on theoretical ethical scenarios such as whether it is right to give liver transplants to alcoholics or to provide surgery to obese patients. On occasions, such discussions may be based on newspaper articles that candidates will have been given either earlier on in the day or sent by email/post several days prior to the interview.

We will deal with all those topics substantially within this book.

1.2 Practical interview stations

Practical interview stations may include activities such as the following:

- **Written task/questionnaire**
  Candidates may be presented with questions that they will need to answer in writing before the "proper" interview starts. In the past, questionnaires have included questions such as "Why do you want to be a doctor" or "Why this medical school?" Questions are rarely different to those that candidates may be asked in a normal interview anyway, and are designed to test candidates' written skills in an environment where they can't get external support (unlike with the personal statement).

- **Discussion around a newspaper article**
  Candidates are presented with a newspaper article (either on the day or sent before the interview) and need to answer questions on issues raised. The articles usually refer to recent ethical issues that have been covered by the press extensively.

- **Communication role play**
  Candidates may be asked to demonstrate how they would communicate with another individual using a role play format. This may include supporting a friend in need, breaking bad news to a friend, a family member or a neighbour, or explaining a task or procedure to another person.

- **Critique of a video doctor-patient consultation**
  Candidates are shown a short video of a medical consultation (usually a GP in a consultation with a patient) and are asked to comment on various aspects of that consultation, e.g. how the GP communicated with the patient, how some of the GP's actions or words impacted on the patient, etc.

- **Group discussion**
  Candidates are placed in small groups (the number of candidates per group can be anything from four to nine) and are given a specific topic to debate in a given amount of time (which can be up to 30 minutes). They are then assessed not only on their personal contribution to the

debate, but also on the manner with which they interacted with the rest of the group.

- **Group task**
  Candidates are placed in small groups to perform a joint task. They are then assessed on their ability to work well within the group and on their ability to ensure that the group reaches the desired outcome.

- **Prioritisation exercise**
  Candidates are presented with a list of tasks that cannot usually all be done at the same time. They then need to determine how they would ensure that all tasks get done within the imposed timescale. Alternatively, candidates may be given a list of objects that they will need to take on holiday with them, only to be told that they cannot pack all of them; they then need to explain how they would choose which ones to leave and which ones to take.

- **Data analysis exercise**
  Candidates are given a paper to read before entering the interview room. The paper usually contains information contained in the form of tables or graphs, but may also contain wordy information. Candidates are asked to answer questions requiring them to draw conclusions from the data given.

This book will help you understand the purpose of those different practical stations and will give you the tools and techniques you need to perform well.

2 Selection criteria

2.1 Different criteria, but one main fundamental set

Different medical schools describe their selection criteria in different ways. Here are a few examples (valid as at publication date):

Hull York Medical School

- Knowledge and understanding of problem-based learning
- Motivation for Medicine
- Depth and breadth of interests, knowledge and reflection about medicine and the wider world
- Teamwork and work experience
- Personal insight – knowledge of own strengths and weaknesses
- Understanding of the role of medicine in society
- Tolerance of uncertainty and ambiguity

UCL Medical School

- Intellectual ability (intellectual curiosity and robustness)
- Motivation for (and understanding of) a career in medicine
- Awareness of scientific and medical issues
- Ability to express and defend opinions, including discussion of BMAT essay topic
- Attitude, including flexibility and integrity
- Individual strengths (e.g. social, musical, sporting interests or activities)
- Communication skills (verbal and listening)
- Following the interview the recommendations of the interviewers

Brighton & Sussex Medical School

- Academic achievement and potential
- A realistic attitude to medical training and clinical practice
- A commitment to caring for others
- The ability to communicate and work effectively within a team
- The ability to appreciate other people's point of view
- Willingness to accept responsibility

St George's Medical School

- Academic ability and intellect
- Empathy
- Initiative and resilience
- Communication skills
- Organisation and problem solving
- Teamwork
- Insight and integrity
- Effective learning style

St Andrew's Medical School

- Empathy
- Good communication and listening skills
- Leadership skills and the ability to work in a team
- A well-informed understanding of what a career in Medicine involves
- Commitment to Medicine by organising work experience or shadowing. Working with ill, disabled, or disadvantaged people, preferably in healthcare settings
- Commitment to academic study, staying power, perseverance and intellectual potential
- Non-academic achievement: positions of responsibility, organisational ability, interests and hobbies, cultural and sporting activities and achievements, social involvement.

Regardless of the wording used by each medical school, those criteria always relate in one way or another to the same fundamental criteria, which are as follows:

Academic ability and intellect
- Appropriate knowledge base and ability to apply judgement
- Ability to manage time and information appropriately
- Capacity to prioritise workload, to balance urgent and important demands and to follow instructions
- Ability to learn effectively both individually and with others

Initiative, resilience and ability to cope with pressure
- Ability to make judgements under pressure
- Awareness of own limitations
- Capacity to demonstrate initiative and resilience to cope with changing circumstances
- Understanding of the need for work-life balance

Communication skills, empathy and sensitivity
- Capacity to communicate effectively and sensitively to others
- Ability to explain ideas in a way that is adapted to the audience
- Capacity to adapt language to the needs of the situation
- Ability to build rapport, to listen, to influence and negotiate
- Capacity to take in others' perspective and treat others with understanding

Problem solving and decision making
- Capacity to use logic and lateral thinking to solve problems and make decisions
- Ability to think beyond the obvious, with a flexible mind
- Capacity to bring a range of approaches to problem solving
- Effective judgement and decision making skills

Managing others, leadership and team playing
- Capacity to work effectively with other people and demonstrate leadership where appropriate
- Capacity to establish good working relations with others
- Ability to support and motivate others

Insight and integrity
- Ability to recognise own mistakes, and learn from them
- Capacity to recognise own limitations and seek advice/help
- Capacity to accept feedback constructively and learn from it
- Ability to deal effectively with criticism

2.2 Why those criteria?

Medical schools want to recruit candidates who can cope with the demands of medical school and of the medical profession, and can become good doctors in accordance with the *Duties of a Doctor* published by the General Medical Council (GMC), which we have reproduced below:

Patients must be able to trust doctors with their lives and health. To justify that trust, you must show respect for human life and you must:

Make the care of your patient your first concern

Protect and promote the health of patients and the public

Provide a good standard of practice and care
- Keep your professional knowledge and skills up to date
- Recognise and work within the limits of your competence
- Work with colleagues in the ways that best serve patients' interests

Treat patients as individuals and respect their dignity
- Treat patients politely and considerately
- Respect patients' right to confidentiality

Work in partnership with patients
- Listen to patients and respond to their concerns and preferences
- Give patients the information they want or need in a way they can understand
- Respect patients' right to reach decisions with you about their treatment and care
- Support patients in caring for themselves to improve and maintain their health

Be honest and open and act with integrity
- Act without delay if you have good reason to believe that you or a colleague may be putting patients at risk
- Never discriminate unfairly against patients or colleagues
- Never abuse your patients' trust in you or the public's trust in the profession

You are personally accountable for your professional practice and must always be prepared to justify your decisions and actions.

BACKGROUND

KNOWLEDGE

At your interview, you may be asked questions that are easier to answer if you possess a little bit of factual knowledge, such as:

- What was the biggest contribution to medical advancement in the history of Medicine?

- How does Medicine now compare to Medicine 200 years ago?

- A 14-year-old girl comes to your surgery asking for contraception. What are the issues?

- What are the current issues facing the NHS?

- How long does it take to train as a consultant or a GP?

In this section, we have set out essential information that will make your job easier on the day. Bear in mind that your interviewers do not expect you to be an expert in the history of Medicine or in ethics. However, they would expect you to have a degree of awareness.

Therefore, do not waste time learning everything in detail and by heart but make sure you are able to use some of that information within your answers in an appropriate manner.

3 A brief history of Medicine

3.1 The birth of Medicine

A long, long time ago ...

In the distant past, Medicine often consisted of a few remedies made from plants, animal parts and crushed minerals, and were often administered by priests and self-appointed medicine men.

Spiritualism (i.e. invoking gods or spirits) was common, as was shamanism (the idea that an individual could cure you by entering a trance and using mystic powers).

Imhotep

It is of course difficult to pinpoint exactly how and through whom Medicine was born, as it was most likely an evolutionary process involving many people across many years. However, Egyptian records show that Imhotep (approx. 2600 BC) was the first recorded physician in history. Imhotep was an important figure in Ancient Egyptian Medicine, having authored a medical treatise remarkable at the time for making no use of magical thinking. This treatise (the so-called Edwin Smith papyrus) contained anatomical observations, ailments and cures.

The cases contained within the Edwin Smith Surgical Papyrus concern:

- 27 head injuries
- 6 throat and neck injuries
- 2 injuries to the clavicle
- 3 injuries to the arm

- 8 injuries to the sternum and ribs
- 1 tumour & 1 abscess of the breast
- 1 injury to the shoulder
- 1 injury to the spine

3.2   The rationalisation of Medicine with Hippocrates

The Greek physician Hippocrates (c. 460–370 BC) is considered by most to be the father of Medicine, principally because he laid the foundation for a rational approach to Medicine. He dismissed the idea that illness could be mystical, preferring to explain disease as the product of environmental factors, diet and living habits. His theories were, however, based on what is now known to be incorrect anatomy and physiology, including the concept of humorism, a theory which stated that the human body was filled with four basic substances, called humours, which are in balance when a person is healthy. The four humours were black bile, yellow bile, phlegm and blood. All diseases and disabilities supposedly resulted from an excess or deficit of one of these four humours. These deficits could be caused by vapours that were inhaled or absorbed by the body. This theory dominated the Western world for over 1300 years.

Hippocrates and his followers were first to describe many diseases and medical conditions. He is given credit for the first description of clubbing of the fingers, an important diagnostic sign in chronic suppurative lung disease, lung cancer and cyanotic heart disease. For this reason, clubbed fingers are sometimes referred to as "Hippocratic fingers".

Hippocrates is of course most famous for setting out the duties and responsibilities of a doctor, in what is known as the Hippocratic Oath, a translation of which is reproduced on the next page. The Oath introduces:

- The notion of free access to care
- The principle of beneficence (acting in the interest of the patient)
- The principle of non-maleficence (not harming the patient)
- The principle of confidentiality

Understandably, the Hippocratic Oath is now outdated and, as such, modern doctors no longer swear it; but many of its principles remain valid today and it forms the premise of the General Medical Council's *Good Medical Practice*[1] and *Duties of a Doctor*[2] (see Section 2.2).

---

[1] http://www.gmc-uk.org/guidance/good_medical_practice.asp
[2] http://www.gmc-uk.org/guidance/good_medical_practice/duties_of_a_doctor.asp

The Hippocratic Oath

Apollo Physician and Asclepius and Hygieia and Panacea and all the gods and goddesses, making them my witnesses, that I will fulfil according to my ability and judgment this oath and this covenant:

To hold him who has taught me this art as equal to my parents and to live my life in partnership with him, and if he is in need of money to give him a share of mine, and to regard his offspring as equal to my brothers in male lineage and to teach them this art - if they desire to learn it - without fee and covenant; to give a share of precepts and oral instruction and all the other learning to my sons and to the sons of him who has instructed me and to pupils who have signed the covenant and have taken an oath according to the medical law, but to no one else.

I will apply dietetic measures for the benefit of the sick according to my ability and judgment; I will keep them from harm and injustice.

I will neither give a deadly drug to anybody if asked for it, nor will I make a suggestion to this effect. Similarly I will not give to a woman an abortive remedy. In purity and holiness I will guard my life and my art.

I will not use the knife, not even on sufferers from stone, but will withdraw in favour of such men as are engaged in this work.

Whatever houses I may visit, I will come for the benefit of the sick, remaining free of all intentional injustice, of all mischief and in particular of sexual relations with both female and male persons, be they free or slaves.

What I may see or hear in the course of the treatment or even outside of the treatment in regard to the life of men, which on no account one must spread abroad, I will keep to myself holding such things shameful to be spoken about.

If I fulfil this path and do not violate it, may it be granted to me to enjoy life and art, being honoured with fame among all men for all time to come; if I transgress it and swear falsely, may the opposite of all this be my lot.

3.3 The Roman Empire

One of the supporters of humorism was the famous Roman physician of Greek descent Galen of Pergamon (*c*. AD 129–200), personal physician to several emperors and recognised as one of the greatest surgeons of the ancient world, having performed brain and eye surgery (his cataract removal technique was not dissimilar to that used by modern day ophthalmologists).

Galen made use of direct observation, dissection and vivisection. He had a strong interest in human anatomy. Since Roman law had prohibited the dissection of human cadavers since about 150 BC, he performed anatomical dissections on living (vivisection) and dead animals, mostly focusing on pigs and primates. This work turned out to be particularly useful because, in most cases, the anatomical structures of these animals closely mirror those of humans.

Galen clarified the anatomy of the trachea and was the first to demonstrate that the larynx generates the voice. He was also the first to recognise that there were distinct differences between venous (dark) and arterial (bright) blood, explained the difference between motor and sensory nerves and discussed the concept of muscle tone.

The Romans were the first civilisation to introduce a true public health system. Rome had grown in size and it became harder to find fresh water, to dispose of rubbish and evacuate used water. As a result, they built many aquaducts to bring water into the city, built public baths to ensure everyone could wash regularly at very low cost, set up an underground sewage system and built public lavatories flushed by fresh clean water. They also drained marshes to get rid of malaria-carrying mosquitoes.

3.4 The Middle Ages

In the Middle Ages (from AD 750), all works written by the fathers of Medicine were translated into Arabic and used by Islamic physicians as a premise to medical research. Physicians such as Muhammad ibn Zakariyā Rāzī (commonly known as Rhazes) (AD 865–925) started querying the validity of the humorism theory (though it remained in place far longer after his death). Rhazes was a prolific author, having written over 200 books, and is credited for being the first to differentiate smallpox from measles and for the discovery of numerous compounds and chemicals including alcohol. He also introduced the notion that even highly educated doctors did not have the answers to all medical problems. He advised practitioners to keep up with advanced knowledge by continually studying medical books and exposing themselves to new information.

The Middle Ages also witnessed the introduction of hospitals, and of medical schools, drawing on the learning of Greek and Arab physicians. In the Mediaeval period the term "hospital" encompassed hostels for travellers, dispensaries for the poor, clinics and surgeries for the injured, and homes for the blind, lame, elderly and mentally ill. Monastic hospitals developed many treatments, both therapeutic and spiritual. Hospitals began to appear in great numbers in France and England. Following the French Norman invasion into England, the explosion of French ideals led most mediaeval monasteries to develop a hospitium or hospice for pilgrims. This hospitium eventually developed into what we now understand as a hospital, with various monks and lay helpers providing the medical care for sick pilgrims and victims of the numerous plagues and chronic diseases that afflicted mediaeval Western Europe. It is thought that the notion of hospital as we know it is a French invention, but that it was originally developed for isolating lepers and plague victims, only later undergoing modification to serve the pilgrim.

The 14th and 15th centuries also saw a major shift in medical thinking, with the rejection of the "traditional authority" approach to Medicine, whereby if someone in authority had said something in the past then it had to be true, in favour of a more evidence-based approach.

3.5 The 16th and 17th centuries

During the Renaissance period, academically trained doctors were particularly important in cities with universities. Medical faculties at universities figured prominently in defining medical guilds and accepted practices as well as the required qualifications for physicians. University-educated physicians and other practitioners were organised according to a strict hierarchy, with university educated physicians on top, followed by learned surgeons; craft-trained surgeons; barber surgeons, who combined blood-letting with the removal of "superfluities" from the skin and head; itinerant specialists such as dentists and oculists; empirics; midwives; clergy who dispensed charitable advice and help; and, finally, ordinary family and neighbours.

Each of these groups practised Medicine in their own capacity and contributed to the overall culture of Medicine, sometimes in very dubious ways. For example, the retention of the humorism theory meant that practices such as blood-letting, using leeches, which would have done more harm than good to a patient, were common. Barber surgeons, who were better at cutting hair and trimming beards than at performing surgical interventions, would not always achieve the desired result, particularly in a world without anaesthetics or antibiotics. Incidentally, the reason why modern surgeons are called Mr and not Dr is because, traditionally, most surgeons were simple barbers as opposed to educated physicians.

The 16th and 17th century nevertheless witnessed significant advances.

Leonardo da Vinci (1452–1519) also had a large impact on medical advances during the Renaissance. Da Vinci's approach to science was based on detailed observation. He participated in several autopsies (mainly on convicted criminals) and created many detailed anatomical drawings, planning a major work of comparative human anatomy.

The Italian Girolamo Fracastoro (1478–1553) suggested that epidemic diseases might be caused by objects outside the body that could be transmitted by direct or indirect contact. He also proposed new treatments for diseases such as syphilis.

In 1543 the Flemish Scholar Andreas Vesalius wrote the first complete textbook on human anatomy. Much later, in 1628, William Harvey explained the circulation of blood through the body in veins and arteries. It was previously thought that blood was the product of food and was absorbed by muscle tissue.

During the 16th century, Paracelsus discovered that illness was caused by agents outside the body such as bacteria, not by imbalances within the body.

The French army doctor Ambroise Paré, born in 1510, revived the ancient Greek method of tying off blood vessels. After amputation the common procedure was to cauterise the open end of the amputated appendage to stop the haemorrhaging. This was done by heating oil, water or metal and touching it to the wound to seal off the blood vessels. Paré also believed in dressing wounds with clean bandages and ointments, including one he made himself composed of eggs, oil of roses and turpentine. He was the first to design artificial hands and limbs for amputation patients. On one of the artificial hands, the two pairs of fingers could be moved for simple grabbing and releasing tasks and the hand looked perfectly natural underneath a glove.

The Englishman William Harvey (1578–1657) accurately described the circulation of blood around the body, and found that the blood was pumped around the body by the heart. Later, the physicians Richard Lower (1631–1691) and Robert Hooke (1635–1703) showed through experimentation that the blood "picked up something" on its way through the lungs, which turned its colour to bright red (it is only in the 18th century, the French chemist Lavoisier discovered oxygen). Lower also performed the first blood transfusion from human to human.

The Dutchman Anton van Leeuwenhoek (1632–1723) invented the microscope and went on to discover red blood cells, bacteria and protozoa. In Italy, physiologist Marcello Malpighi (1628–1694) used the microscope to study the structure of the liver, spleen, lungs, skin, glands and brain. Several microscopic parts of the body (e.g. a skin layer and parts of the spleen and kidney) are named after him.

The Englishman Tomas Willis (1621–1675) discovered the presence of sugar in the urine of diabetics and was a pioneer in research into the anatomy of the brain, nervous system and muscles. He coined the term "neurology" and documented the anatomy of the brain and nerves in minute detail. He was the first to number the cranial nerves in the order in which they are now usually enumerated by anatomists.

3.6 The 18th century

The 18th century was a great century for advances in diagnostics. The Dutch professor Hermann Boerhaave (1668–1738) started making systematic use of the thermometer to monitor body temperature and the Austrian physician Leopold Auenbrugger (1722–1809) discovered the need to tap on the chest to look for fluid in the lungs.

The 18th century also saw great advances in therapeutics. The English surgeon James Lind (1716–1794) proved that scurvy (a vitamin C deficiency disease) could be cured by eating citrus fruit. The botanist William Withering (1741–1799) showed the effectiveness of digitalis in treating heart diseases. A British country doctor Edward Jenner (1749–1823) developed the smallpox vaccine, which was so successful that smallpox has now been eradicated (the word "vaccination" comes from the Latin "vacca" meaning "cow" because the smallpox vaccine was developed from liquid taken from cow pox lesions).

However, despite a wealth of discoveries, there was a huge gap between those new discoveries and the practice of Medicine on the ground. The main treatments still remained cupping, bleeding and purging, following the old Greek tradition. Syphilis was treated with massive (and often fatal) doses of mercury. Many of the physicians were reluctant to adopt new ideas and "serious" physicians such as William Harvey even stated that they had lost patients as a result of adopting new techniques.

In the early 1700s, the French physician Pierre Fauchard started dentistry science as we know it today. In 1761, veterinary Medicine was properly separated from human Medicine when the French veterinarian Claude Bourgelat founded the world's first veterinary school in Lyon, France. Before this, medical doctors treated both humans and animals.

Background knowledge

3.7 The 19th century

Cell theory

After much faltering, medical practice finally began to change in the 19th century. A major improvement to the workings of microscopes made it possible to study tissues and cells in more detail, leading to the new science of cells called cytology. Cell theory, which states that all living things are made up of cells that are the basic unit of structure and are produced from other cells, is one of the cornerstones of modern Medicine. Using cell theory, the German scientist Rudolf Wichrow (1821–1902) demonstrated that changes in cells can cause diseases such as cancer.

Germ theory

Another cornerstone of modern Medicine, which stems from the 19th century, is germ theory. In the past, some advocates of humoral Medicine had recognised (contrary to their beliefs) that some diseases may have been spread by contagion. Some Muslim scholars had already attributed the bubonic plague to microorganisms. However, generally speaking, most physicians believed that diseases-causing germs appeared spontaneously, a belief which lasted from Aristotle (c. 350 BC) to the 19th century. However, all that changed when the English physician John Snow (1813–1858) traced the source of cholera to water contaminated by sewage.

Shortly thereafter, the French chemist Louis Pasteur ran a series of experiments which concluded that life could not be spontaneously generated. Pasteur demonstrated that there were in fact organisms everywhere in the air (through an experiment which turned milk sour) and went on to develop a process that heats milk to kill microbes, now known as pasteurisation. His further work on microorganisms also led him to develop vaccines against anthrax and rabies.

Germ theory was firmly implanted within Medicine by a German physician named Robert Koch (1843–1910) who identified the specific bacteria that caused anthrax, tuberculosis and cholera, and developed a set of postulates (rules) to help ascertain conclusively whether a microorganism was the source of a disease as opposed to simply being present. This was the beginning of the science of bacteriology (or microbiology).

Anaesthesia

Back in the 16th century, a Swiss-born physician commonly known as Paracelsus made chickens breathe sweet vitriol and noted that they not only fell asleep but also felt no pain. Later in 1730, a German chemist called Frobenius gave the liquid the name "ether" which is Greek for "heavenly". But it would not be used as an anaesthetic until 1842, being used commonly from 1846 onwards. Drawbacks with ether such as excessive vomiting and its flammability led to its replacement in England by chloroform.

Discovered in 1831, the use of chloroform as an anaesthetic is linked to James Young Simpson, who found chloroform's efficacy in 1847. Its use spread quickly and gained royal approval in 1853 when John Snow gave it to Queen Victoria during the birth of Prince Leopold. Unfortunately, chloroform is not as safe an agent as ether, especially when administered by an untrained practitioner (medical students, nurses and, occasionally, members of the public were often pressed into giving anaesthetics at this time). This led to many deaths from the use of chloroform that (with hindsight) might have been preventable.

Antiseptics

In the middle of the 19th century, a Hungarian physician Ignaz Semmelweiss (1818–1865) discovered that infections in obstetrics units following childbirth were most likely due to poor hand-washing by physicians. In the late 1860s, the British surgeon Joseph Lister (1827–1912) helped greatly reduce the rate of death from gangrene by dipping bandages and ligatures into carbolic acid and pouring the acid into the wounds to sterilise them. This marked the start of antiseptic surgery.

3.8 The 20th century

A huge boost in pharmacology

Towards the end of the 19th century, huge efforts were invested to understand the chemical composition of plants and synthesise drugs. For example, aspirin (a synthesised version of acetylsalicylic acid) was first isolated by Felix Hoffmann, a chemist with the German company Bayer, in 1897.

In 1909, the German scientist Paul Ehrlich (1854–1955) synthesised the arsenic-based compound Salvarsan, the first effective treatment for syphilis, thus creating the first antibiotic. In 1928, Alexander Fleming spotted mould growing on some bacterial samples in his laboratory and, as a result, discovered penicillin. Tests carried out during World War II showed that it was effective against anthrax, tetanus, syphilis and pneumonia. However, penicillin proved hard to mass produce and, as a result, was not widely available until 1944.

In 1943, an American biochemist isolated streptomycin, which proved effective against tuberculosis.

Other notable discoveries included:

- Vaccines against tetanus (1925, with 2 new vaccines in 2005); influenza (1933), smallpox and polio (1950s, leading to the eradication of polio by the end of the 20th century), measles (1963), chickenpox (1995), human papillomavirus vaccine (causing cervical cancer) (2006)
- Cortisone, a steroid hormone to reduce inflammation and suppress the immune system response (1950s)
- The contraceptive pill (1960s)
- Chlorpromazine for psychoses, lithium carbonate for mania (1950s), and then, in rapid succession, the development of tricyclic antidepressants, monoamine oxidase inhibitors and benzodiazepines, among other antipsychotics and antidepressants

The first antiviral drug, acyclovir, appeared in the 1970s to combat herpes. The 1980s saw the development of antiretroviral drugs to combat AIDS.

The rise of technology

Imaging: At the very end of the 19th century, in 1895, the German physicist Wilhelm Conrad Röntgen (1845–1923) discovered X-rays, making it possible to look at the internal organs of the body. In 1901, a Dutch physiologist Willem Einthoven (1860–1927) invented the first electrocardiograph. Further inventions came later, enabling physicians to observe the body in a non-intrusive manner. These included:

- Ultrasound imaging (1949)
- Computerised tomography or CT scan (1970s)
- Positron-emission tomography, or PET scan (1975)
- Magnetic resonance imaging or MRI scan (late 1970s)

Surgery: In the mid 20th century, the heart-lung machine was developed, providing artificial means to keep patients alive whilst surgeons operated on the stopped heart. This cardiopulmonary bypass made major heart surgery more routine. The 1970s saw the invention of flexible endoscopes, allowing the introduction of laparoscopic surgery (commonly referred to as keyhole surgery). In such operations, the endoscope, which carries a camera and a laser, is inserted into a tiny incision. This is commonly used for procedures on hernias, gall bladders, kidneys and knees.

Artificial organs: The poor availability of organs for transplant has encouraged the development of artificial organs. The first artificial kidney (for use in haemodialysis) was invented in 1913, allowing life prolongation for patients with kidney failure. Artificial hearts were first implanted in 1982.

Prosthetics: Though artificial limbs have existed for some time (the oldest surviving examples date back to 300 BC), the discovery of plastic in the mid-20th century, and of other advanced material such as carbon fibre, has enabled the creation of devices that operate by electronic attachment to the muscles. The latest devices are controlled by microchips.

Computers: Computers have made a huge contribution to medical advancement. Not only do they play a key role in scanning technology, they also run the machines in surgical theatres and intensive care units. Medical records and prescriptions can be handled electronically, research data could not be analysed without computers, and mapping the human genome would not have been possible without the vast power that computers offer.

A better understanding of the immune system

Immunisation (i.e. vaccination) was practised in Ancient China and brought to the West by Edward Jenner. However, no one until the 20th century understood the science behind it.

In the 1880s, the Russian biologist Elie Metchnikoff (1845–1916) discovered phagocytosis after experimenting on the larvae of starfish. He realised that the process of digestion in microorganisms was essentially the same as that carried out by white blood cells. His theory, that certain white blood cells could engulf and destroy harmful bodies such as bacteria, met with scepticism from leading specialists including Louis Pasteur, Behring and others. At the time most bacteriologists believed that white blood cells ingested pathogens and then spread them further through the body. Less than two decades later, Paul Ehrlich (1854–1915) argued that the chief agents of immunity were, in fact, antibodies, i.e. proteins produced by cells and released into the bloodstream. In the end both theories turned out to be correct but the enormous complexities of the immune system continue to be unravelled to this day.

Progress in immunology also included the identification of a class of disorders called autoimmune diseases (whereby the body is basically attacking itself), such as Type-1 diabetes, lupus, muscular dystrophy and rheumatoid arthritis, and a range of drugs to go with them (called immunosuppressants). These immunosuppressants also play a vital role in ensuring that transplant patients are able to retain the organs that were transplanted, thus making organ transplantation an almost routine procedure, and ensuring that virtually any organ of the body can be transplanted from one person to another (subject to availability of course). Immune therapy also offers hope in the fight against some cancers.

The identification of the HIV virus in the 1980s brought the science of immunology back to the fore. The HIV virus destroys the immune system and therefore the body's ability to respond to threats. Though there is, to date, no cure for HIV/AIDS, there now exists a range of treatments that help patients reach a normal life expectancy. AIDS is no longer the death sentence it used to be.

The quest for an AIDS vaccine is still ongoing; it is one of the most vexing in all of science because, unlike other viruses, HIV mutates frequently to outmanoeuvre antibodies that fight against it.

31

A rise in genetics

The vast majority of the progress made in immunological and viral studies is due to a new understanding of genetics.

Though DNA had been isolated by the Swiss physician Friedrich Miescher (1844–1895) in 1869, its structure was decoded in 1953 by British bio-chemist Francis Crick (1916–2004) and American biologist James Watson (born 1928). Knowledge of the DNA structure made it possible to determine the location of each gene. By the early 21st century, scientists had mapped the genetic structure of humans (so-called human genome).

Cracking the genetic code also enabled the introduction of testing for diseases caused by defective chromosomes such as cystic fibrosis, Huntington's disease and some forms of breast cancer. It has also enabled the creation of new drugs derived from natural body chemicals such as insulin and human growth hormone.

From a genetic perspective, the greatest avenue of research is gene therapy, which would enable the curing of diseases by inserting normal copies of abnormal genes directly into cells by means of a virus. Progress so far has, however, been very limited.

4 The NHS

4.1 Healthcare in the UK before the NHS (pre-1948)

The 16th to the 19th centuries

There has been some form of state-funded provision of health and social care in England for 400 years. Historically, the poor, infirm and elderly received care from religious orders, particularly the monasteries. In 1543, King Henry VIII established himself as head of a newly-created Church of England, in order to legitimise his second marriage to Anne Boleyn. England was subsequently excommunicated from the Catholic Church and, in return, the King dissolved the monasteries, removing the main source of care for vulnerable people.

Over the next 50 years, various measures were introduced to support those with the greatest need. In 1601, under Queen Elizabeth I, these were brought together under the first Poor Law. This established almshouses to care for the poor and sick, and a system of "outdoor relief", providing benefits in kind to support the poor at home. Outdoor relief was assistance, in the form of money, food, clothing or goods, given to alleviate poverty without the requirement that the recipient enter an institution. In contrast, recipients of "indoor relief" were required to enter a workhouse or poorhouse. This remained the main source of state-sponsored care until the 19th century. By then, attitudes towards the poor had changed and the care provided by almshouses was thought to be too benevolent. Outdoor relief was abolished and austere workhouses were established, providing accommodation for the poor, orphans and the elderly. Although the different groups were supposed to be looked after separately, in practice this rarely happened and everyone was housed in single, large institutions. Towards the end of the century, annexes were added to house the sick. Care was rudimentary, often provided by untrained volunteers, and Florence Nightingale, amongst others, commented on the atrocious conditions. Until then nurses had mostly been religious, monastic women or untrained helpers of low repute.

The 20th century

By the 20th century, as the pathological basis of disease became better understood, healthcare was increasingly provided by other bodies. A network of charitable and voluntary organisations and local and municipal authorities established hospitals. Charitable and voluntary hospitals dealt mainly with serious illnesses, rather than long-term care. Medical care was provided by visiting specialists who had lucrative private practices elsewhere.

Most beds were provided in municipal hospitals by the local authorities of counties and large towns from the rates (taxes) as a service to their ratepayers. Local authorities also provided maternity hospitals, hospitals for infectious diseases (scarlet fever, smallpox and tuberculosis), and institutions for the elderly, mentally ill and handicapped and a variety of community services. The standard varied widely, depending upon the attitude of the council.

Bed rest was a major form of treatment for heart attacks, ulcers, tuberculosis and childbirth. Lengths of stay could be several weeks.

A quarter of hospital beds were provided in voluntary hospitals. These varied from small hospitals supported by public subscription, to internationally famous teaching hospitals such as St Bartholomew's, Guy's and St Thomas', which received significant investment income. Some hospitals were developed in conjunction with universities – University College Hospital, King's College Hospital and the provincial teaching hospitals. Special hospitals concentrated on particular diseases or types of patients, children or women. But each voluntary hospital was a law unto itself, raising funds and deciding its admission policies. In London, the King's Fund had, since 1897, attempted to bring some order to the financial accounts, management, the location of voluntary hospitals, and to help with their costs. Patients were often charged and many hospitals were near bankrupt.

Mentally ill people

Mentally ill people were generally sent away to large forbidding institutions, not always for their own benefit, but because that was how the system worked. Admission was often for life. Under the poor conditions prevailing, many patients became worse rather than better and "institutionalised". There was, however, a basic standard of food and accommodation.

Older people

Older people who were no longer able to look after themselves fared particularly badly. Many ended their lives in the Public Assistance Institutions, the old workhouses feared by everyone. Workhouses changed their names in 1929, but their character and the stigma attached to them remained. One of the early achievements in the NHS was the development of geriatrics, which tackled the problem of the "back wards", seldom visited by doctors, where people ended their days.

Community services

Primary and community care services evolved separately from the hospitals. Community care, environmental and public health services were the responsibilities of local authorities. In 1911, the government, under Lloyd George, passed the National Insurance Act. This funded a family doctor service for all working men on low pay, enabling them access to a GP from a "panel" of local doctors, free of charge. This "panel system", although not providing cover to wives, children or their dependants, made a considerable difference to a large proportion of the poor, entitling them to free, government-funded healthcare. "Panels" were often operated by Friendly Societies that paid GPs as little as possible. Outside the scheme, medical treatment had to be paid for – often according to what the patient could afford. GPs in affluent areas could rely on income from their patients. In 1919 the Ministry of Health was established and a Scottish Board of Health created to improve public health and to encourage research, treatment and medical training.

In the First World War the army medical services had shown the benefits of organisation and transport. At the government's request, in 1920, Lord Dawson produced a forward-thinking report on how a health service might be organised. Under the Local Government Act (1929) local authorities took over poor law hospitals, which became municipal hospitals serving ratepayers, not paupers. They needed much upgrading. The quality varied widely from town to town and rural areas were poorly served. Some areas had duplicated services and others had minimal specialist services.

Drivers for change

There was a bipartisan agreement that the existing services needed to be improved. The main drivers for change included the following:
- The emergence of a view that healthcare was a right, not something bestowed erratically by charity
- Financial difficulties for the voluntary hospitals
- The impact of the war made it possible for transformation of the system, rather than incremental modification
- An increasing view among the younger members of the medical profession that there was a better way of doing things.

The first step in creating a nationalised health service took place in 1938. The imminent war obliged the government to establish an Emergency Medical Service. All types of hospitals were registered, funded and run centrally to prepare for large numbers of expected casualties.

In 1942, the Beveridge Report described a vision for welfare reform based on eradication of the five giants of: idleness, squalor, hunger, disease and ignorance.

A major issue that later split the Labour Party was whether a future NHS should be run by local authorities, or quite separately on a regional basis. During the war the Conservatives produced the first White Paper on a health service led by local authorities.

The coalition government's 1944 White Paper stated the aims of the new health service:

> "to ensure that, in future, every man and woman and child can rely on getting all the advice and treatment and care which they may need in matters of personal health; that what they get shall be the best medical and other facilities available; that their getting these shall not depend on whether they can pay for them, or any other factor irrelevant to the real need."

After Labour's election victory in 1945, the Health Minister, Aneurin Bevan, presented to the Cabinet a radically different plan favouring nationalisation of all hospitals, voluntary or council, and a regional framework. After much tough negotiation this plan went through, with modest concessions.

In 1948, the NHS was finally born.

4.2 Overview of NHS provision of care today

The NHS was founded in 1948 based on the three following principles:

1. That it met the needs of everyone
2. That it be free at the point of delivery
3. That it be based on clinical need, and not ability to pay.

Those three principles still hold true on the whole. However, since then some services are now incurring charges; many people have to pay for prescriptions in England and Northern Ireland (Wales and Scotland have free prescriptions for everyone), for dental services and for optical services.

Across the whole of the UK, healthcare is provided using a GP gateway (or hierarchy) model. This means that, with the exception of walk-in services such as Accident & Emergency (A&E) or Genito-Urinary Medicine (GUM), patients need to go first to a GP before being granted access to a specialist service.

Primary care

The term "primary care" refers to the first point of contact in the healthcare system. In the NHS, the main source of primary healthcare is general practice. The aim is to provide an easily accessible route to care, whatever the patient's problem. Primary healthcare is based on caring for people rather than specific diseases. This means that professionals working in primary care are generalists, dealing with a broad range of physical, psychological and social problems, rather than specialists in any particular disease area.

The best-known providers of primary care services are General Practitioners (GPs). An important role of GPs is acting as the patient's advocate and coordinating the care of the many people who have multiple health problems. Since primary care practitioners often care for people over extended periods of time, the relationship between patient and doctor is particularly important. Primary healthcare involves providing treatment for common illnesses, the management of long-term illnesses such as diabetes and heart disease, and the prevention of future ill health through advice, immunisation and screening programmes. When necessary, GPs refer patients to specialists working in secondary care.

GPs usually work in practices with other GPs, though it is estimated that single-handed GPs (i.e. GPs working on their own) care for about 5m patients in total in the UK. GPs are not employed by the NHS. They (or their practice) are effectively proper businesses, which are contracted to provide services to NHS patients. Because of that, they are responsible for providing adequate premises from which to practise and for employing their own staff. A typical GP practice will include GP partners (those who own the practice) and salaried GPs (who are simply employed to provide a service to the practice).

Secondary care

The term "secondary care" refers to care provided by medical specialists and other health professionals who generally do not have first contact with patients and for which you may need to be referred by a GP. This would include, for example, cardiologists, urologists and dermatologists. It is generally provided in hospitals (though there are exceptions, such as psychiatry). It may be unplanned emergency care or surgery, or planned specialist medical care or surgery. Patients are usually referred to secondary care specialists by their GP.

Tertiary care

The term "tertiary care" refers to super-specialised care provided by health professionals to patients referred to them by a secondary care health professional. This includes cancer management, neurosurgery, cardiac surgery, plastic surgery, treatment for severe burns, advanced neonatology services, palliative care, and other complex medical and surgical interventions. Tertiary care is normally provided only in teaching hospitals or other specialist hospitals.

Quaternary care

The term "quaternary care" refers to care which is so specialised that only a few people with very rare problems will ever need it. It covers experimental medicine as well as uncommon diagnostic and surgical procedures. For that reason there are not many quaternary care services.

Example of referral pathway from primary to tertiary care

Primary care
A patient comes to the GP after a fit. After obtaining information from the patient about the nature of the fit, the GP suspects that the patient may have epilepsy. He refers the patient to a neurologist.

↓

Secondary care
The neurologist sees the patient, carries out some tests and prescribes appropriate medication. However, after 2 years, the patient is not fully stable and the neurologist feels that he needs to see a neurologist specialising in epilepsy.

↓

Tertiary care
The neurologist with special interest in epilepsy is able to use his more specific knowledge to pinpoint the exact nature of the problem, and addresses it successfully.

In many instances, problems can be solved by the GP without the need to refer a patient to secondary care. In many instances too, if a patient needs to be referred to secondary care, there is no need for him/her to be referred to tertiary care specialists.

So, although this system may mean that a patient has to wait a little longer to see the specialist they need, it also ensures that the time of those specialists is not wasted on simple cases that can be dealt with at a lower level.

4.3 The NHS in England

Commissioning of services

In England, each hospital essentially operates as an independent business. The decision as to which healthcare provider is allowed to provide which services is made by Clinical Commissioning Groups (CCGs), which consist mainly of local GPs and managers (with a few representatives from hospitals). So, for example, a local CCG may decide that Hospital X should no longer provide hip replacement surgery, because from now on such surgery should be provided by Hospitals Y and Z only.

Legislation that came into effect in 2013 has made it possible for external providers (e.g. charities or even private companies) to offer NHS services. So, for example, a local CCG could decide to award a contract for cataract surgery to a private company rather than to the local hospital (though of course they would need to have a good reason to do that: a good reason being that they feel the private company may provide better quality of care). The process of awarding contracts is known in the NHS as "commissioning".

Because CCGs are local groups and consist mainly of GPs, they cannot commission GP services themselves. Similarly, they can't commission services that need to be provided on a more global scale because of their specialist nature, such as heart and lung transplant surgery or eye cancer care for two reasons:

1. They don't have the skills and knowledge to understand the exact nature of those services.

2. Those services are provided on a regional or national basis.

Instead, both primary care services and specialist services are commissioned by a higher body, which used to be called the NHS Commissioning Board but is now known simply as NHS England.

Block Contract vs. Payment by Results

Before 2005, hospitals were paid a fixed amount of money every year, designed to cover the cost of healthcare. That system was called "block contract". If a hospital needed more money (i.e. was in deficit compared to their budget), then the government would simply pay more money to that hospital. Conversely if a hospital spent less money (i.e. showed a profit against its budget) then it would have to pay it back to the government. The problems with that approach were that there was no incentive for hospitals to save money or work efficiently.

In 2005, the Labour government introduced the principle of "Payment by Results", whereby a tariff would be set nationally for each clinic and each procedure. Hospitals would no longer receive a fixed amount of money but would instead be paid for each activity they undertook. So, for example, a hip replacement might have a tariff of £5,000, which would cover the cost of the hospital stay, imaging, the surgery and some follow-up. The amount of the tariff would be set roughly at the average of the cost across all trusts, meaning that some hospitals would make a loss and others would make a profit. The idea was to encourage those who made a loss to work more efficiently so that they could make a profit and survive.

The main problem with "Payment by Results" when it was introduced was that it ensured that hospitals were paid for what they did and that they were encouraged to perform efficiently, but it did not encourage hospitals to provide quality of care. Action therefore needed to be taken so that hospitals did not just focus on making a profit but also provided quality care to patients. Such actions included:

- Giving patients the choice of where they wanted their care to be provided, whereby the GP would give patients a list of hospitals to which they could go, and the patient would then choose the place that suited them most: the hope being that patients would make the choice on the basis of the quality of care they expected to receive.

- Imposing targets that had to be reached (for example max 4-hour wait in A&E, max 18-week wait for elective surgery).

- Ensuring that hospitals were penalised for poor quality care (for example by ensuring that, if a patient had to be readmitted to hospital following a complication of the surgery, the hospital would have to deal with that complication without expecting to be paid).

- Introducing incentives to provide enhanced standards of care. For example, the NHS introduced a sort of bonus scheme called CQUIN (Commissioning for Quality and Innovation) which rewards departments that enhance the quality of care of their patients. GPs were encouraged through a sort of bonus scheme too (called QOF – Quality of Outcomes Framework). In addition, hospitals that succeeded in providing best practice care to their patients could benefit from higher tariffs in some specialities.

- Increasing competition between healthcare providers (see below).

The role of the private sector in the provision of healthcare

When it comes to the private sector, the issues can appear complicated and confusing. There are several ways in which the private sector is involved and, although, you will not need to know any of this in much detail, you must know enough to understand what part of the private sector an interview question is referring to before you can answer it. The different types of private providers are as follows:

1. *Private practice doctors (referred to as "private healthcare"):* this normally refers to doctors working for private hospitals or for themselves who provide healthcare to individual private patients. Examples of private healthcare providers include BUPA or AXA PPP. These private providers have been around for a long time and are normally used by patients to bypass the NHS waiting lists. Patients either pay for the care themselves or through a private healthcare insurance company. The doctors involved in private healthcare are often the same as those working for the NHS, who undertake private activities in their spare time. The prices charged by those private providers are subject to market forces and are typically way higher than the standard NHS tariff for the same procedures.

   So, for example, if a patient has been told that they would need to wait 4 months to get a hip replacement on the NHS but wants it earlier, that patient can go to a private orthopaedic surgeon who will perform the operation a lot sooner. The patient will then have to pay with their own money unless they have private insurance. In exchange they can expect more attention from staff, their own private room and a guarantee to be seen by a consultant.

2. *External (i.e. non-NHS) providers contracted to do NHS work:* this refers to private companies, charities or other organisations who have been officially commissioned to provide healthcare to NHS patients at NHS tariffs. An example of this is Virgin Care who provides services to NHS patients in areas as diverse as breast cancer screening, paediatric physiotherapy, sexual health services or dermatology clinics. Those services are commissioned by the CCGs, and are provided at no direct cost to the patient. Basically this is NHS care provided at NHS tariffs by non-NHS providers.

It is the introduction of those private providers contracted to do NHS work that has led many to fear a "privatisation of the NHS". Here are the arguments commonly presented for and against such a system (which we have tried to present in as balanced a way as possible):

- Private companies are run for profit. There is a risk that they will therefore favour making profits over providing quality care. The counter-argument to this is that the NHS has been run on a not-for-profit basis for many years and has not always provided the best quality care it could (see later the section on the Mid-Staffordshire Trust). In addition, though there is some anecdotal evidence that some private companies engage in dubious practices or do not deliver in line with expectations, this is not widespread (and again the NHS has its own share of dubious practices too).

- Private companies may "cherry-pick" the easy cases that are the most profitable, leaving the NHS burdened with the more complex, loss-making cases. The answer to that argument is that it is, indeed, true for the simple reason that one would not want those private companies to take on complex cases they can't handle. Those companies would be asked to handle the simple high volume work to ensure that that work is being done efficiently without interference from other work such as emergencies; it follows then that the NHS (with more expertise than the private sector) should handle the more complex cases that it has been trained to handle well. The reason NHS trusts may be losing money on those more complex cases is because the tariffs have not been calculated well enough to ensure they can cover their costs. However, it is a matter of time before this anomaly is resolved.

- "Privatisation" will lead to fragmentation of care. If different aspects of care are given to different providers then healthcare may be provided in many more venues than under the old system (where basically care was only provided either in a GP practice or in a hospital). This may mean that patients will have to travel to different places in order to be seen, which will cause issues with patient records, for example, since there is no central database that can be accessed from everywhere.

- The fragmentation of care described in the previous paragraph will also lead to training issues. External providers will be handling the simple cases, which are those used as part of medical training. A private company that needs to make a profit may be reluctant to train doctors if that leads to a loss of profit.

- There are risks of conflict of interest amongst doctors. Many of those external providers are, in fact, at least partially owned by doctors. For example, many out-of-hours services are owned by GPs. Some hospital consultants have also set up external businesses, which could be competing against the same hospital trust in which they work. The commissioning of such services therefore has to be done in an open and transparent manner.

4.4 The NHS in Wales, Scotland and Northern Ireland

Wales

The reorganisation of NHS Wales, which came into effect on 1st October 2009, created single local health organisations that are responsible for delivering all healthcare services within a geographical area, rather than the Trust and Local Health Board system that existed previously. The reorganisation abolished the internal market. There are seven Health Boards. In Wales, healthcare funding is still based on block contracts between Welsh commissioners and the relevant providers. Funding to hospitals from Welsh commissioners is therefore based on historical activity and funding levels as a guide for the expected number of treatments over the coming year. Clinical activities are not funded on the basis of actual activities provided. Instead, an overall figure of anticipated activity is agreed in advance between the commissioner and the provider.

The Health and Social Services budget is £6 billion, 40% of the Welsh Assembly's total budget. From 1st April 2007 the NHS prescription charge was abolished for people in Wales.

Scotland

The Scottish Government Health Directorate (SGHD) has responsibility for NHS Scotland as well as the development and implementation of community health policy. The SGHD undertakes the central management of NHS Scotland and heads a Management Executive that oversees the activity of the 14 area NHS boards. The roles of the Health Boards include strategic leadership and performance management of the entire local NHS system in their areas and assurance that services are delivered safely, effectively and cost-efficiently. The 14 NHS Boards are ultimately responsible for the commissioning, provision and management of the full range of health services in an area including Hospitals and General Practice.

Payment to hospitals is on a block contract basis. Like Wales, Scotland offers free prescriptions to its residents. The budget for NHS Scotland is £11 billion, just over one-third of the Scottish Government's annual budget.

Northern Ireland

In Northern Ireland the National Health Service is referred to as HSC or Health and Social Care. Just like the other NHS it is free at the point of delivery but in Northern Ireland it also provides social care services such as home care services, family and children's services, day care services and social work services.

The Department of Health, Social Services and Public Safety has overall authority for health and social care services. Services are commissioned by the Health and Social Care Board and provided by five Health and Social Care Trusts – Belfast, the largest of the five, South Eastern, Southern, Northern and Western.

The Health and Social Care Board sits between the Department and Trusts and is responsible for commissioning services, managing resources and performance improvement. Inside the Board there are Local Commissioning Groups (LCGs) focusing on the planning and resourcing of services. The LCGs cover the same geographical areas as the five Health and Social Care Trusts.

The budget for the Department of Health, Social Services and Public Safety is £4 billion, 40% of the Northern Ireland Executive's annual budget.

4.5 Key bodies

The General Medical Council (GMC)

The GMC has four distinct roles:

- Keeping a register of all qualified doctors. In practice no doctor can practise in the UK without being registered with the GMC.

- Fostering good medical practice. It does so by issuing guidance on standards that doctors need to adhere to, such as *Good Medical Practice,* the modern equivalent of the Hippocratic Oath, and by ensuring that doctors are regularly revalidated.

- Promoting high standards of medical education and training. The GMC sets and monitors standards for post-undergraduate and post-graduate trainees. It also provides guidance to ensure that doctors are supported in their continuing professional development.

- Dealing with doctors who may not be fit to practise. Those doctors are investigated and in some cases may be suspended or struck off from the medical register.

The Royal Colleges

Royal Colleges are institutions charged with setting standards within their field and for supervising the training of doctors within that specialty. Most of them grant membership to doctors only once they have passed a number of examinations. For example, trainees who want to get into surgery will need to pass the MRCS (Membership of the Royal College of Surgeons) examinations.

Existing colleges include:

- Royal College of Surgeons of Edinburgh (RCSEd)
- Royal College of Physicians of London (RCP)
- Royal College of Physicians and Surgeons of Glasgow (RCPSG)
- Royal College of Physicians of Ireland (RCPI)
- Royal College of Physicians of Edinburgh (RCPE)
- Royal College of Surgeons of Ireland (RCSI)

- Royal College of Surgeons of England (RCS)
- Royal College of Obstetricians and Gynaecologists (RCOG)
- Royal College of General Practitioners (RCGP)
- Royal College of Pathologists (RCPath)
- Royal College of Psychiatrists (RCPsych)
- Royal College of Radiologists (RCR)
- Royal College of Ophthalmologists (RCOphth)
- Royal College of Anaesthetists (RCoA)
- Royal College of Paediatrics and Child Health (RCPCH)
- College of Emergency Medicine (CEM) (This one is not Royal!)

The British Medical Association (BMA)

The BMA is essentially the trade union representing doctors. Unlike the GMC and Royal Colleges, membership is not compulsory.

Medical Defence Union (MDU) / Medical Protection Society (MPS)

The MDU and the MPS are the two largest defence unions for doctors. Their role is to insure doctors against lawsuits and to represent them in court or in a GMC hearing. They also provide educational activities for their members.

National Institute for Health and Care Excellence (NICE)

NICE is an independent organisation providing guidance on health promotion and the prevention and treatment of ill health. It provides guidance in the following areas:

- Health technologies, i.e. which new or existing medicines, medical devices, procedures, diagnostic techniques or treatment should be used within the NHS. NICE makes recommendations as to which medicine, investigations, devices or procedures should be used, not only on the basis of their effectiveness but also on the basis of cost. NICE focuses on the principle of "value for money". NICE therefore plays an important role in the rationing of drugs, treatments and investigations in the NHS.

- Interventional procedures: in essence, NICE assesses the safety of a range of procedures and provides information about their safety. It can then recommend a procedure for routine use or specify any special steps that should be taken when seeking consent from patients for the least safe procedures. These guidelines are different to other guidelines as they are mostly informative rather than prescriptive.

- Clinical practice, i.e. which treatments are appropriate for people with specific diseases or conditions. NICE also produces guidelines that are designed to improve the quality of care of patients with specific conditions or diseases. These clinical guidelines are based on the best available evidence but do not replace the clinician's judgement, which still needs to be exercised. They can therefore be considered as "a guide that should be followed unless there is a good reason not to do so".

- Public health: the Centre for Public Health Excellence (part of NICE) publishes guidelines on nine different areas: smoking and tobacco control; obesity, diet and nutrition; exercise and physical activity; alcohol; sexual health; mental health; drug misuse; promoting the health of children and young people; preventing accidental injury. The guidance can provide advice on the amount and level of information that should be given to the population on these key areas; it can also take the form of recommendations on strategies to address key issues such as smoking cessation or teenage pregnancies.

Care Quality Commission (CQC)

The independent regulator of all health and social care services in England, the Care Quality Commission inspects hospitals, care homes, GP surgeries, dental practices and other care services to ensure they meet national standards of quality and safety.

Monitor

Monitor is a regulator looking after the health of the finances of NHS trusts. It regularly assesses NHS trusts to ensure they are well led, in terms of both quality and finances.

5 Key issues and topics you need to know about

5.1 Harold Shipman

Harold Shipman was practising as a GP in the Manchester area and was convicted of the murder of 15 patients and of forging a will, although it is alleged that he actually murdered hundreds of his patients, mostly by injecting opiates (morphine, etc.) into their body.

Shipman had started to experience blackouts 4 years after graduating from medical school and, although it was first thought to be due to epilepsy, it transpired that he had, in fact, an opiate addiction. He was convicted and fined £600 for this. He was also barred from taking up any job that would give him access to controlled drugs. At this point the GMC did not take any steps to strike him off the Medical Register.

In 1977 he took up a post as a GP in Hyde and, although regarded as arrogant by his colleagues, he was well regarded by his patients. In 1992 he left his practice to set up on his own, taking with him a long list of patients. In 1997 staff at a funeral parlour started to become suspicious at the high number of deaths from elderly people who did not seem to be particularly ill prior to their death. Their death had either been certified by Shipman or followed a recent visit by Shipman. A rival GP surgery also became suspicious. As a result, the police were notified but were unable to reach any conclusions.

Nothing more happened until the daughter of one of the victims became concerned at the fact that her mother had left her possessions to her GP and launched an enquiry about the possible forgery of the will. This resulted in Shipman being charged and convicted of 15 murders and forgery; the other murders were not investigated thoroughly as Shipman had already been jailed for life anyway and many of the alleged victims had been cremated, which made any enquiry difficult.

In 2001 Dame Janet Smith conducted an enquiry into the murders and concluded that 215 deaths could be attributed to Shipman, 45 were most likely murdered by Shipman (but this was only a strong suspicion) and 38 cases could not be proven due to insufficient evidence.

Consequences of the Shipman case

The Shipman case led to a number of changes directly or indirectly. In particular:

1. **A move away from single-handed GP practices.** As Shipman was working on his own, there were few opportunities for colleagues to check on what he was doing. As a result, he was able to murder many people without questions being asked.

2. **Tighter regulations on the use of controlled drugs.** Not only was Shipman able to get hold of controlled drugs despite an earlier conviction, he was also able to get hold of large quantities to murder hundreds of patients.

3. **Tighter regulation of death certification.** Shipman managed to get many patients cremated, which required two signatures (one by him and one by another doctor). There was failure on the part of these other doctors to recognise the situation. There are now plans to report all deaths to a coroner. This would introduce an additional degree of scrutiny, though it may overburden coroners.

4. **Review of the revalidation process**, which ensures that doctors have the necessary skills to practise. It was recognised that there had been a failure on the part of the GMC to deal with Shipman when it could have made a difference. Obviously, hindsight is always easy to invoke, but the GMC was criticised at the time for acting too much in the interest of doctors and not enough in the interest of patients. Ultimately, it must also be recognised that no amount of bureaucracy will ever prevent a murderer from operating, though it may make it easier to stop one in his tracks at an early stage (rather than wait for 200 murders). See Section 5.4 for more details on revalidation.

5.2 MMR vaccination and the 2013 measles epidemic

In 1998, a surgeon called Andrew Wakefield published a research paper showing that there was a link between the administration of the Measles, Mumps and Rubella (MMR) vaccine and the development of autism and bowel disease. At a press conference and in a video news release issued by the Royal Free Hospital NHS Trust, he called for suspension of the triple MMR vaccine until more research could be done. He suggested parents should opt for single jabs against measles, mumps and rubella, separated by gaps of one year.

Several issues, however, arose, which discredited the research carried out. In particular:

1. No other researchers were able to confirm the results found by Andrew Wakefield.

2. A Sunday Times reporter produced documentary evidence that Wakefield applied for a patent on a single-jab measles vaccine before his campaign against the MMR vaccine, raising questions about his motives. Wakefield – in partnership with the father of one of the boys in the study – had planned to launch a venture on the back of an MMR vaccination scare that would profit from new medical tests and "litigation driven testing". *The Washington Post* reported that Deer said that Wakefield predicted he "could make more than $43 million a year from diagnostic kits" for the new condition – autistic enterocolitis.

3. One of Wakefield's former students testified that Wakefield ignored laboratory data that conflicted with his hypothesis.

4. The research was based only on 12 cases, which Andrew Wakefield claimed were previously normal but 5 had, in fact, documented pre-existing developmental concerns.

5. Some children were reported to have experienced first behavioural symptoms within days of MMR, but the records documented these as starting some months after vaccination.

Between 2007 and 2010, the GMC investigated the allegations and concluded that Andrew Wakefield:

- Was being paid to conduct the study by solicitors representing parents who believed their children had been harmed by MMR.

- Ordered investigations "without the requisite paediatric qualifications" including colonoscopies, colon biopsies and lumbar punctures ("spinal taps") on his research subjects without the approval of his department's ethics board and contrary to the children's clinical interests, when these diagnostic tests were not indicated by the children's symptoms or medical history.

- Acted dishonestly and irresponsibly in failing to disclose how patients were recruited for the study. In particular it came to light that he had purchased blood samples for £5 each from children present at his son's birthday party, which Wakefield joked about in a later presentation.

- Conducted the study on a basis that was not approved by the hospital's ethics committee.

As a result he was struck off the UK Medical Register in May 2010.

The measles epidemic

As a result of Andrew Wakefield's statements and a reporting failure by most media (the public wasn't getting a balanced view from the media, as it wasn't reporting some of the robust studies in 1999 and 2000, which showed there was no causal link between MMR and autism), many parents around the world became worried that their children may develop autism as a result of MMR vaccination and decided against giving the MMR vaccine to their children, with some parents opting to give individual vaccines instead or no vaccine at all. It was reported that immunisation rates in Britain dropped from 92% to 73%, and were as low as 50% in some parts of London. According to the Centers for Disease Control and Prevention in the United States, more cases of measles were reported in 2008 than any year since 1997. More than 90% of those infected had not been vaccinated, or their vaccination status was not known.

In Wales in March, April and May 2013, over 1200 people became infected with measles as a result of a lack of vaccination, leading to an urgent MMR vaccination campaign.

5.3 The structure of medical training

The structure of medical training varies between specialties. Within each specialty, trainees may also take slightly different paths, meaning that some may take longer than others to train if they decide to undertake training activities beyond the scope of the normal syllabus or research activities.

On the whole, the post-medical-school training system works as follows:

Step 1: Foundation Years (FY)

After leaving medical school, every trainee doctor without exception undertakes 2 years of Foundation Training. Those 2 years are designed to help young doctors get used to working as "proper" doctors and ensure that they acquire a sound basis for their future training. During that period, doctors are called FY1 and FY2.

Step 2: Core Training (CT)

Core Training years are designed to give trainees a good basis in their area of interest.

All those who wish to work in a medical specialty (e.g. cardiology, respiratory medicine, renal medicine, oncology, genito-urinary medicine, etc.) must undertake 2 years of Core Medical Training (CMT), which is common to all medical specialties.

All those who wish to work in a surgical specialty (e.g. cardiothoracic surgery, general surgery, ear nose and throat, etc.) will undertake 2 years of Core Surgical Training, or CST.

Whilst core training for Medicine and surgery can lead to many different specialties, some specialties have their own core training. For example psychiatry has a 3-year core training period, which is only for psychiatry.

During the core training years, doctors are called CT1, CT2 (and CT3 if relevant). Once a doctor has gone through his core training grades, he can apply for specialist training (ST) through a competitive process (usually application form + interview).

Step 3: Specialist Training (ST)

The duration of Specialist Training ranges from 4 to 9 years. For a specialty such as genito-urinary medicine or emergency medicine, specialist training is 4 years only. However, for a specialty such as ear, nose and throat, this could be as long as 9 years. In cardiology, the specialist training lasts 5 years.

During those years, doctors are called ST3, ST4, etc.

Variations for run-through specialties

Some specialties such as paediatrics, obstetrics & gynaecology, ophthalmology and radiology do not require a core training period before taking on trainees at specialist level. For those specialties, Core Training and Specialist Training is basically merged into one large period, meaning that trainees don't always need to apply to new posts in the middle of their training. That is why they are called run-through training schemes. Once you are in, you are in.

Example of training pathways

Paediatrics
- 2 years of Foundation Programme (FY1-FY2)
- Application form + interview
- 8 years run-through Specialist Training programme (ST1-ST8)

Psychiatry
- 2 years of Foundation Programme (FY1-FY2)
- Application form + interview
- 3 years of Core Training in psychiatry (CT1-CT3)
- Application form + interview
- 3 years of Specialist Training (ST4-ST6)

Cardiology
- 2 years of Foundation Programme (FY1-FY2)
- Application form + interview
- 2 years of Core Medical Training (CT1-CT2)
- Application form + interview
- 5 years of Specialist Training (ST3-ST7)

Trauma & Orthopaedics
- 2 years of Foundation Programme (FY1-FY2)
- Application form + interview
- 2 years of Core Surgical Training (CT1-CT2)
- Application form + interview
- 5 years of Specialist Training (ST3-ST7)

(Note that, in Scotland, recruitment into Trauma & Orthopaedics takes place straight after the 2 Foundation Years, i.e. it is run-through training.)

Time needed to become a consultant

The shortest training programmes after the two Foundation Years are in Public Health, Clinical Radiology, Clinical Pathology and Microbiology/Virology, which last 5 years and have no core training.

One of the longest training schemes is Ear Nose & Throat, which can take up to 9 years on top of the 2 Foundation Years and the 2 Core Surgical Training years.

It can therefore take 7 to 13 years before someone fresh out of medical school can become a consultant (so on average approximately 10 years), with medical training usually being slightly shorter than surgical training. However, this does not take into account any additional training or experience that doctors may wish to acquire. For example, some doctors may want to take time out to carry out research activities; if they undertake a PhD, this could add a further 3 years to their training. Other doctors decide to go on a specialist fellowship (e.g. spend a year in Australia or the US to learn a particular technique); fellowships are up to a year long. In some specialties, some may undergo several fellowships in a row.

GP training

Approximately 50% of doctors who qualify train to become GPs. The training currently consists of 3 years of General Practice training following the two Foundation Years. The training usually consists of 2 years in hospitals and 1 year in general practice. One can therefore become a GP 5 years following the end of medical school. There are talks to increase GP training time from 3 years to 4 years, making it 6 years in total.

See www.medicalcareers.nhs.uk for more information on medical training.

5.4 Revalidation

The origins of revalidation

The idea of revalidation arose many years ago as the result of several medical scandals. The idea was to find a system that would impose regular checks on doctors to ensure that they are fit to practise. The aim of revalidation is to protect patients from poorly performing doctors, promote good medical practice and, generally, increase public confidence in doctors.

Under the original pre-2000 proposals, doctors would have submitted records of appraisals, including personal development plans and feedback. They would also have submitted CPD records. Based on that evidence the GMC would have decided whether to revalidate a doctor or insist on further action.

The 5th Shipman report and suspension of revalidation

Following the Shipman affair (see Section 5.1), an enquiry was conducted by Dame Janet Smith into the various components of the scandal. This included an enquiry into the role of the GMC, which resulted in the so-called 5th Shipman Report. The report essentially criticised the GMC for looking after doctors more than after patients and for not taking reasonable steps to protect patients by revalidating doctors properly. It also highlighted the poor sharing of information on doctors' performance between the professional, educational and regulatory bodies. The GMC's role was also criticised, particularly the fact that it sets the rules, investigates doctors and passes judgement on their actions.

When the GMC was criticised for letting Harold Shipman kill hundreds of victims unnoticed, it defended itself by presenting revalidation as the answer to the problem.

The Shipman case mainly concerned a failure by the NHS to audit Shipman's activities in a number of areas including:

- Cremation forms (and a second signature more or less applied without checks).

- A high mortality rate amongst his patients (all of whom were elderly and whose deaths were simply dismissed as unlucky or natural).

- A discrepancy in the prescription of diamorphine and other controlled drugs (all the more bizarre since Shipman had already been suspended by the GMC for stealing drugs in the 1970s).

It was established that Shipman was well liked by colleagues and patients, and that therefore he would have passed appraisals with flying colours. He also kept up to date and would have had no problem being revalidated on the basis of those two criteria alone. As a result, the GMC had no choice but to suspend revalidation (before it was even fully introduced) and to go back to the drawing board.

Revalidation at last! (Late 2012)

After much thinking and deliberation, the GMC finally came up with a solution for revalidation. Revalidation started on 3 December 2012, with the majority of licensed doctors in the UK expected to revalidate for the first time by March 2016. Revalidation consists of regular appraisals with the employer, based on *Good Medical Practice*.

- Licensed doctors are required to link to a Responsible Officer.

- Licensed doctors need to maintain a portfolio of supporting information drawn from their practice, which demonstrates how they are continuing to meet the principles and values set out in the *Good Medical Practice* Framework for appraisal and revalidation.

- Licensed doctors are expected to participate in a process of annual appraisal based on their portfolio of supporting information.

- The Responsible Officer will make a recommendation to the GMC about a doctor's fitness to practise, normally every five years. The recommendation will be based on the outcome of a licensed doctor's annual appraisals over the course of five years, combined with information drawn from the clinical governance system of the organisation in which the licensed doctor works.

- The GMC's decision to revalidate a licensed doctor will be informed by the Responsible Officer's recommendation.

The portfolio needs to contain the following information:

1. **General information** such as personal details, scope of work, record of annual appraisals, personal development plans and their review, statement on probity and health.

2. **Continuous Professional Development record,** i.e. record of courses and conferences attended, journals read, etc.

3. **Review of own practice** including quality improvement activities such as clinical audit, review of clinical outcomes or case review; and description of significant events.

4. **Feedback on own practice** including colleague and patient feedback, as well as a review of complaints and compliments.

Pros and cons of revalidation

Pros	Cons
<ul><li>Formalises practices that may have been done on an ad hoc basis previously.</li><li>Ensures compliance with some basic requirements and provides focus to the appraisal process.</li></ul>	<ul><li>Will not stop another Shipman</li><li>Senior clinicians may see it as their way to fulfil their management responsibilities and may consequently not ensure proper management of individuals at other periods of the year.</li><li>Runs the risk of identifying underperformance only at the "once-a-year appraisal point", i.e. in some cases too late.</li><li>The process may require information that trusts do not hold (e.g. for surgeons, individual results).</li></ul>

5.5 Clinical governance

Clinical governance is a concept familiar to all doctors (or at least it should be). It is essentially a set of principles and behaviours that all doctors should adhere to in order to ensure that they offer their patients the best quality clinical care. The realm of clinical governance is comprehensive but here are some of its fundamental principles:

1. Doctors should ensure that their practice is compliant with the latest evidence. They should keep up to date and should ensure that they constantly adjust their practice to match new guidelines and new evidence from research. They should also formally audit their adherence to guidelines and best practice (see Section 5.6).

2. Doctors should provide safe care to their patients and ensure they do not place their patients at risk (e.g. they must make sure they wash their hands appropriately, check the drugs they prescribe, etc.). They should feel comfortable owning up to their mistakes and learning from them. They should report any incident so it can be investigated and lessons can be learnt.

3. Doctors should ensure that they recognise when they have reached their limitations and should be willing to ask for help when necessary. Similarly, if doctors come across colleagues whose practice may endanger patients, they should act upon it and raise those issues with someone senior.

4. Doctors should ensure they constantly develop their skills and should also train and educate others. All staff should be properly supported.

5. Doctors should be attentive to patient needs and should take account of feedback they receive from members of the public to ensure they constantly improve their services.

5.6 The audit process

Audits are a systematic examination of current practice to assess how well an institution or a practitioner is performing against set standards. Essentially, it is a method for reflecting on, reviewing and improving practice. Audits are a fundamental part of the duties of doctors and ensure that all doctors and departments are compliant with guidelines, protocols and best practice standards.

How does an audit work?

The audit process is often referred to as the "audit cycle", essentially because it is a continuous loop. The process is as follows:

1. Choose a topic for the audit, i.e. a practice to be investigated.
2. Define a standard that you would like to achieve.
3. Collect relevant data.
4. Compare results of analysis against standard.
5. Identify changes that need to be made in order to reach standard.
6. Implement changes and give time for those changes to be fully operational.
7. Re-audit (complete the loop) several months later to measure the impact of the changes.

Why are audits important?

- The main purpose of an audit is to identify weaknesses in your practice and increase the quality of service provided to users.

- Audits also help to identify inefficiencies and ultimately may lead to a better use of resources.

- Audits are also used to provide information about quality of care to outside agencies, for the production of league tables, etc.

- Audits provide opportunities for training and education.

5.7 The Mid-Staffordshire NHS Foundation Trust scandal

Many patients and relatives of patients who had attended Stafford Hospital were very unhappy at the care (or lack of care) they had received. A local campaign group "Cure the NHS", led by a relative whose mother died at the hospital, campaigned for an enquiry. Between 2009 and 2013 a series of enquiries were conducted, which revealed an astonishing story of poor care and negligence.

The Healthcare Commission report (2009)

The report highlighted a series of failures particularly in A&E, Acute Medical Unit and on some medical and surgical wards. Those concerns related to:

- Poor nursing standards
- Lack of effective management systems for emergencies
- Failure to identify and act on high mortality rates for patients admitted as emergencies
- A Board detached from day-to-day reality of patient care
- Failure by the Board to develop an open culture and to challenge current practice despite information pointing to obvious problems.

The report qualified the care received by patients as "appalling" and mentioned that this likely led to hundreds of unnecessary deaths. Between 400 and 1,200 more people died than would have been expected in a 3-year period from 2005 to 2008, the Commission said.

The first Francis enquiry (2010)

The first enquiry was designed to identify key failures and make recommendations. Led by Robert Francis QC, it identified a "bullying culture, target focused in which the needs of the patients were ignored" and "an appalling failure at all levels". Key failures identified included:

Board failures
- The Board buried its head in the sand, failed to appreciate the enormity of the issues, reacted too slowly and generally downplayed the significance of many of the issues identified. For example, the chief executive had concluded that high mortality rates were due to coding issues.

- The Board responded to the Healthcare Commission report with denial. It showed no lack of urgency to resolve the issues raised.
- Too much focus was placed on finances (the trust had been making losses for a few years). To save £10m (8% of its turnover), the trust set out to make cuts, including removing 150 posts. Wards were badly reorganised (separate floors for surgery and Medicine without carrying out any risk assessment), beds were cut and consequently patient care was compromised.
- Poor governance (clinical audit practice underdeveloped, critical incidents not reported or not acted upon, investigation of complaints done by staff from the area which caused the problem in the first place (and not seen by the Board)).

Staff-related issues
- Too few consultants and nurses.
- Constant change of management, leading to lack of leadership.
- Doctors isolated from managers, the Board and each other.
- Some key individuals were unsafe.
- Lack of attention to patient dignity (incontinent patients left in degrading conditions, patients left inadequately dressed in full public view, patients handled badly – sometimes by unskilled staff – causing pain and distress, rudeness, hostility, failure to refer to patients by name).
- Poor communication (lack of compassion and sensitivity, lack of information about patients' condition and care, lack of involvement of patients in decisions, friends and family often ignored, failure to listen and reluctance to give information, staff not communicating well with each other, wrong information provided to patients and relatives).
- Poor diagnosis and management (slow or premature discharge of patients, discharge from A&E without appropriate diagnosis or management, poor record keeping, poor or delayed diagnosis).
- Buzzers left unanswered.

Cultural issues
- Patients concerned about insisting on proper care for fear of upsetting staff or of reprisals.
- Staff distracted by their own mobile phones.
- Staff not focussed on basics (litter left on the floor, alcohol gel not replenished and therefore not used).
- Low staff morale.

The second Francis enquiry (2013)

The second enquiry focused on commissioning, supervision and regulation of the hospital, querying particularly why such serious issues were not identified earlier and acted upon sooner. The enquiry highlighted the following issues:

Cultural issues
- Blame culture not eradicated.
- Defensiveness and secrecy.
- Complacency towards poor standards.
- Failure to put patients first.
- A degree of bullying.

Stakeholders
- Doctors failed to speak up for patients.
- PCTs and SHAs had blind trust in the hospital's management and accepted their reassurance without further checks.
- Monitor and CQC did not challenge enough.
- The Royal College of Nursing was not supportive enough of its members when they raised concerns.
- Department of Health too remote.
- GPs did not raise concerns until after the issues came to light.

Amongst the 290 recommendations the report made, here are some of the key ones:

- There should be more focus on compassion and caring in nursing recruitment, training and education.
- Patient safety should be the number 1 priority in both medical and nursing training and education.
- Individuals and organisations will have a duty to speak up (the government is, in fact, considering the possibility of criminal prosecution for staff who don't).
- Quality accounts should be published in a common format and made public.
- The profession of healthcare assistants should be regulated.
- For the elderly, one person should be in charge of individual patient care.
- The Royal College of Nurses should be either a royal college or a trade union, not both.
- Patient involvement must be increased.

5.8 The four ethical principles

At an interview, you may be asked questions containing ethical scenarios. Though daunting at first, those questions are actually fairly easy to answer if you are aware of and understand the four ethical principles that underlie medical practice. The four principles are as follows:

Autonomy

Patients are entitled to their opinion and to make decisions for themselves. In particular, patients have the right to choose the treatment that they feel is best for them and also have the right to refuse to be treated. A key factor for this principle to apply is that the patient must be in a position to understand and process the information at his disposal to make an informed decision. This is referred to as "patient competence" (see Section 5.10).

Note that the principle of Autonomy refers to the right that the patient has to accept or to refuse a treatment or procedure that is offered by a doctor. It does not mean that the patient can demand from doctors the treatment that they want. So if, at an interview, you are asked what you would when faced with a patient who demands to be given a particular course of treatment that you know will not be effective, you should not give that treatment. You should only prescribe the treatment that you think would be in the best interest of the patient; the patient can then decide whether to take it or leave it. If there are several options with equal benefits (e.g. surgery vs. medical treatment) then the options should be presented to the patient and the patient can then make an appropriate choice for themselves.

Beneficence

The word comes from the Latin "bene" = "good" and "facere" = "to do". Doctors must "do good" and act in the best interest of their patients.

Non-maleficence

From the Latin "male" = "bad, harmful", this term means that a doctor should act in such a way that he does not harm his patients, whether it is actively or by omission.

Justice (sometimes also called "equity")

Put simply, this is about fairness across the population. Patients who are in the same position should be considered in the same way (i.e. you can only discriminate on the basis of different clinical needs). Benefits, risks and costs should also be spread fairly. This includes taking into account that some resources such as money, time, organs, etc. are in short supply.

Right to confidentiality – the fifth element

Confidentiality is not strictly speaking an ethical principle, but it is linked to some of them. For example, confidentiality can be part of patient autonomy and the right of the patient to control the information that pertains to their own health. Confidentiality can also be linked to non-maleficence in that you may harm the patient by revealing information about them.

Ethical dilemmas originate from the fact that there is a clash between two or more of the above principles. For example, consider the daily decisions that a physician in Intensive Care has to make for a patient who is in great pain and needs large doses of morphine. Giving the patient an increasing dose of morphine helps relieve his pain and is therefore consistent with the principle of beneficence as it is doing good to the patient. However, an increased dose of morphine may also bring the patient closer to his death, thus harming him. Here, the principle of beneficence clashes with the principle of non-maleficence and the physician will therefore need to strike the right balance to act in the best interest of the patient.

5.9   Informed consent

Informed consent means that the patient has consented to a procedure or treatment, having been given and having considered all the facts that were necessary for them to make a decision in their own best interest.

Before a patient can give their consent for a particular procedure, the doctor must explain a number of facts, including:

- Options for treatment or management of the condition (whether this is through surgical or medical management). This includes the option not to give treatment.

- The aim of the planned procedure or treatment, including any consequences, common or serious side effects.

- Details of the planned procedure or treatment, its benefits, chances of success, as well as common or serious risks and side effects, and how these might be managed.

- Consequences of providing the treatment versus consequences of not providing the treatment.

- Details of any secondary interventions that may be required while undertaking the first one (e.g. blood transfusion if heavy blood loss during surgery) and for which the patient should provide consent beforehand as they will be unable to do so should it be required in an emergency.

- Details of who will be performing the procedure and whether doctors in training will be involved (particularly important for surgical interventions).

- A reminder that the patient can change their mind at any time and that they can seek a second opinion.

- Any costs that the patient may incur (mostly relevant for private work).

Following on from this, the patient should be given any appropriate written information such as leaflets explaining the procedure, its risks and benefits. The patient should also be given enough time to reflect so that they do not feel pressured into making a decision.

Only competent patients can give consent. For more details on competence, including seeking consent from children, see Section 5.10.

Note that, in theory, doctors should obtain consent for everything they do. That includes procedures, blood tests and examinations but also simple things such as taking your blood pressure. In practice though, there are many simple tasks for which consent is not explicitly sought, but is taken to be implied.

For example, if a doctor wants to take a patient's blood pressure, he will often take it for granted that the patient has an understanding of what that means. As the doctor approaches the patient and instructs the patient to roll up their sleeves, the fact that the patient actually rolls up their sleeves and presents their arm to the doctor signals that they are consenting to having their blood pressure taken. However, implied consent only really applies to simple tasks with no real consequences. Anything else requires explicit consent to be obtained.

5.10 Competence of a patient

Consent can only be taken from patients who are deemed to be "competent", i.e. who understand the information given to them and are capable of making a rational decision by themselves. Competence is a legal judgement. Doctors also frequently talk about "capacity to consent" or "mental capacity". This is a medical judgement. Capacity is formally assessed by doctors and nurses who must be sure that a patient is able to understand a management course, to comprehend the risks and benefits and to retain that information long enough to make balanced choices. As with competency, capacity is situation and time specific, i.e. a patient may have capacity to decide on a breakfast menu but not on an option for a knee amputation.

The two terms have a similar meaning but in different contexts (legal and medical) and you will find that, for that reason, there is a tendency for people to use them interchangeably. However, it may be useful to understand the distinction between the two, if only to answer a picky interviewer's question on the matter. For our purpose, we will use the word "competent".

Adults

Adults (and children aged 16 and 17) are deemed competent unless proven otherwise. If an adult is not competent, for example because they have a serious mental disorder, no other party can give consent on their behalf. There are two options:

1. If the patient has issued an advance directive (also called "living will") at an earlier date stating how they would wish to be treated if at some point they were no longer able to make decisions for themselves, then doctors would then need to abide by the patient's decision, even if such a decision was not necessarily in their best interest.

2. If the patient has not indicated any particular wishes, the decision will rest with doctors to act in the best interest of the patient. However, doctors should involve relatives in order to ascertain what the patient would have wanted.

Children below the age of 16 (Gillick competence/Fraser guidelines)

Children under the age of 16 are deemed competent to give consent if they are shown to be mature enough to understand the information given to them about the procedure and its consequences. However, the doctor has a duty to discuss with the child the possible involvement of the parents or legal guardian in the discussions. Note that if the child refuses to involve the parents then the doctor will have to respect their decision, as this would otherwise constitute a breach of confidentiality (see Section 5.11 for further details on confidentiality). A doctor will only be able to involve the parents against the will of the child if the child is deemed not to be competent (in which case parental involvement is mandatory) or if the child is in danger (in which case you would involve social services or the police).

These principles are called "Gillick competence" or, more commonly now, "Fraser guidelines" after the name of a complainant and judge respectively in a famous court case. Please note the following:

- The competence of a child is assessed in relation to the procedure concerned. For example, a 5-year-old boy will most certainly be competent for the application of an antiseptic on a small cut, but will not be competent to give consent for the removal of one of his testicles.

- Although a child can give consent for a procedure or treatment if competent, in England and Wales they cannot refuse consent for a procedure or treatment that is deemed in their best interest. For example, if a doctor established that a boy with a form of cancer needed a surgical intervention, the boy would not be allowed to refuse. The decision would need to be made by his parents.

- If both the parents refused to give consent on behalf of their child for a life-saving procedure, doctors would need to act in the best interest of the child. If possible, they should get a court order to impose the treatment. If time is of the essence, they may need to impose the treatment first and justify that decision later in court if needed.

Important note: As mentioned above, children cannot refuse consent for a procedure or treatment. This applies in England and Wales. However, in Scotland, children are allowed to refuse consent.

5.11 Confidentiality

What is the duty of confidentiality?

Except for very specific circumstances addressed below, all doctors should protect the confidentiality of their patients at all costs. Breaching the confidentiality of a patient could have serious consequences for the patient (for example, divulging an illness to a family member) and his trust in the medical profession. It could also prevent the patient from divulging crucial information about his health in future. Ultimately, it would constitute a serious professional fault on the doctor's part and, in extreme circumstances, could lead to the end of his career as a doctor.

When can you breach confidentiality?

1 – Implied consent has been given by the patient

For example, a patient will understand that you need to provide information about them to other members of your team in order to care for them (e.g. nurses, or a hospital consultant if you are referring). However, if a patient explicitly mentions that they do not wish you to share information with a colleague, you must comply with their request and work around it if possible.

Other forms of implied consent include a patient who visits your surgery with a family member and openly discusses their situation with you. However, you must be careful when it comes to disclosing important information. For example, a patient may have brought her husband along but, if you feel that you have to break bad news or deal with a sensitive issue, you will need to check with the patient first.

2 – Information required by a court/judge

For example, if the police need access to medical records in the course of an investigation (insurance fraud, etc.). This requires a court order.

3 – In the public interest and to protect the patient or others

This includes:

- Where the interest to society or others of disclosing the information without the patient's consent outweighs the benefit to the patient of keeping the information confidential.

- Notification to the authorities of notifiable diseases (e.g. meningitis, tuberculosis, mumps, measles, etc. – see www.hpa.org.uk for full list). Note that HIV and AIDS are not notifiable.

- Suspected cases of child abuse or of neglect, physical or emotional abuse, where the patient cannot give consent to disclosure.

- Informing the DVLA if a patient's condition may affect his driving (e.g. diabetes in lorry drivers, epilepsy, etc.).

- When the information can help with the fight against terrorism or in identifying a driver who committed a road traffic offence (though the disclosure should be limited to the strictly necessary data, i.e. often address details and not clinical information).

5.12 Euthanasia & Assisted Suicide

Euthanasia

The word "euthanasia" refers to a situation where someone ends someone else's life through an intentional act in order to alleviate their pain and suffering (the word "euthanasia" means "good death" in Greek). There are two types of euthanasia:

- Active euthanasia, i.e. the act of ending someone's life through a practical action such as poisoning them or suffocating them.

- Passive euthanasia, i.e. where the lack of action results in the death of the person. This would include withholding treatment that may prolong their life (e.g. ventilator, antibiotics).

  Those can be further subdivided between the following categories:

- Voluntary euthanasia, where the person whose life is ended has given their consent.

- Non-voluntary euthanasia, where the person whose life is ended was not able to provide consent (e.g. they were in a vegetative state or unable to communicate, such as a small child).

- Involuntary euthanasia, where the person whose life is ended would have been in a position to give consent, but instead indicated they did not wish to die or were not asked.

Assisted suicide

The term "Assisted Suicide" refers to a situation where an individual essentially commits suicide with the help of someone else. They could be helped, for example, by a doctor who prescribes them medication to induce death, or by a relative who helps them overdose.

The Swiss connection

There are institutions abroad (e.g. Switzerland) where patients can go to receive euthanasia. Following an assessment, patients are injected with a lethal cocktail of drugs, which relaxes them and enables them to die peacefully. Obviously, such a possibility is only open to people who can actually travel there. The decision would need to be taken entirely by the patient and could certainly not be made on the recommendation of a UK doctor (otherwise they would be in breach of the non-maleficence principle).

Arguments in favour of euthanasia and assisted suicide

1. Patients should be allowed to choose what is best for them.
2. Patients can avoid a lengthy and unnecessary suffering period.
3. Patients can die with dignity at a time of their choosing.
4. It would free up beds and other NHS resources utilised for these patients.

Arguments against euthanasia and assisted suicide

1. It goes against some religious principles. It may lead to doctors or relatives playing God.
2. Even if someone has expressed the wish to receive euthanasia when they are in distress, they may change their mind later at a time when they may no longer be able to express their change of position.
3. There have been cases where people, who were in situations where everyone thought they were a lost cause, actually recovered.
4. It would be very difficult to verbalise specific criteria for allowing or disallowing euthanasia/assisted suicide.
5. If the case is not clear-cut or well documented, relatives may face murder charges (e.g. following a complaint by other relatives).
6. Relatives may abuse the situation by allowing convenient euthanasia on a patient to suit their own needs.
7. Relatives may pressure a patient into a situation they do not actually wish.

The legal position

In the UK, both euthanasia and assisted suicide are illegal. Those who commit such acts (they often are carers or relatives who fail to cope with a person's illness or commit mercy killings) are routinely taken to court and often convicted of manslaughter, and occasionally murder.

Some have even been prosecuted for simply making travel arrangements on behalf of a sick relative so that they could travel to a Swiss clinic to die there. There have been several high profile cases of this nature and the police are taking a keen interest in the relatives who travel with the patient. The main argument is that, by accompanying a relative to a so-called "death clinic" (or even by booking a plane ticket for them), they are effectively assisting a suicide, which is illegal. In practice though, such police investigations rarely lead to a conviction, particularly if it can be proven that the patient travelled there of their own free will and the relatives did not play an active role. This is perhaps a sign that society is slowly adapting.

The ethical dilemma for doctors

Doctors may be confronted by situations where they may need to withdraw treatment from an individual: such action potentially leading to the death of the patient. This may happen if the patient is unable to communicate their wishes and the doctors believe that a particular treatment is not effective and is not in the patient's best interest.

In such situations, unless the patient has issued an Advanced Directive stating what should be done in the event that they can no longer communicate, the decision to withdraw treatment rests entirely with the doctors. The relatives do not have the right to make these decisions, although it is best practice for the doctor to consult with them over treatment decisions.

An example that occurs commonly is the decision to undertake cardiopulmonary resuscitation on a patient whose heart has stopped or who has stopped breathing.

FORMAL INTERVIEW STATIONS

Q&A FORMAT

(Applicable to both standard and MMI interviews)

6 Key interview techniques

6.1 Giving meaningful and confident answers

Interviews are all about conveying information in a convincing and confident manner. They are therefore, primarily, a communication exercise. It is important that you understand and respect some key principles, which will enable you to present meaningful and confident answers.

Keep your answers to 1½ to 2 minutes

No one can listen to anyone for more than 2 minutes unless that speaker is absolutely fascinating or has some visual aids to help retain concentration. There is therefore no point in giving answers that are much longer as you run the risk of boring your interviewers.

Conversely, if your answers are too short you will not have the opportunity to give the information the interviewers need to make a decision. You need to explain what you say, back up all your statements appropriately and generally provide a well-developed answer. Therefore your answers should be sufficiently long to be interesting.

On balance, a length of 1½ minutes seems to be what works best, in the knowledge that you can push your answer to 2 minutes if you need to.

Structure your answers well. Stick to 3 or 4 points

Your interviewers will be in the same room for some time, listening to similar answers to the same questions all day long. You must therefore make it easy for them to understand the points that you are trying to communicate. To achieve this, make no more than 3 or 4 points within an answer – this is as much as anyone will be prepared to listen to, and certainly as much as anyone will remember. Raising too many points will simply make you lose your audience. If you have more than a handful of points to make, see if you can reorganise the information into bigger headings.

Make sure that you actually answer the question

Too many candidates talk around the question without answering it. For example, if the question is "What qualities do you have that would make you a good doctor?", a response such as "Well, in my work experience, I really enjoyed talking to the hospice residents and really enjoyed working with the team" does not actually answer the question.

However, "One of my strong points is that I am very empathic and a good team player" is a direct answer to the question. Once you have made your point then you can provide more detail to elaborate on it.

If you feel you really need an introduction, keep it short.

Use facts to substantiate your answers. Give examples

During the course of your interview, you will make many statements which, if not developed well, will sound impersonal and vague. For example "I feel I have all the attributes to be a good doctor", or "I chose my work experience carefully to match my career aspirations." Such statements make good opening sentences but are too vague to convey anything useful to interviewers.

Whenever you make a statement, take some time to explain what you mean and give examples. Facts bring credibility to your answer. You can draw from your work or academic experience to discuss who, what, when, why and how, and to personalise your answers.

Be positive and use power words to sell yourself

Keep the answers positive. Sell yourself. There is no need to volunteer the negative facts. When discussing negative situations, use your answer to explain how much you have learnt from your experience.

Use the passive tense sparsely. "Many skills were developed as a result of that experience" does not sound as good as "I developed many skills as a result of that experience".

Whenever you can, use power words, i.e. words that convey more specifically what you have achieved. For example "During the Young Enterprise project, I worked with my colleagues to secure funding to the tune of

£1,000" sounds a little vague. However, "I produced a marketing plan which enabled the team to raise £1,000" sounds more focused.

In Section 12, you will find a list of 500 power words you may consider using to strengthen your answers.

Talk about yourself rather than everyone else

Candidates who feel uncomfortable at interviews usually compensate by talking about everything else but themselves. An interviewer will hear a lot of sentences of the type "During my Duke of Edinburgh, we did a long walk. That was particularly hard because some members of the team struggled and they had to be supported and motivated." Such a sentence only describes a context but does not explain your role; more importantly it gives no information about the skills that you demonstrated, making it hard for the interviewers to determine whether you would make a good doctor.

Don't talk solely about "the team" or "we". Talk about "I", "my responsibilities", "my aim", etc. If your answer gives good examples and is specific about what you did, you will not sound arrogant.

Only talk about what you know and mind the probing

If you want to mention something into which the interviewers can probe, make sure that you have all the answers. For example:

- If you mention the name of a condition – for example because you came across it during your personal life or your work experience – make sure you know what that condition entails and have some understanding of how it can be managed.

- If you mention a scientific fact – for example you state that stem cells are an interesting area to explore for future development – make sure you can demonstrate the relevant level of knowledge if the interviewers decide to quiz you.

Having said that, if you know a particular topic well, nothing stops you from "involuntarily" dropping it into the conversation, knowing or hoping they might ask you to talk about it. That would be a clever way of seizing control of the conversation.

6.2 How not to sound arrogant

A number of people who are perfectly normal in real life end up sounding arrogant at interview. Even those who don't sound arrogant are worried that they might come across as braggers. Consequently, in an effort to remove any trace of possible arrogance from their answers, candidates tend to play their achievements down ("we achieved a lot as a team"), introduce self-deprecation ("I think I am a good communicator but I am sure that there are many things I can improve on), or depersonalise their answers ("a lot was achieved during that time"). This makes them sound vague, uninteresting and impersonal, which is possibly worse than sounding arrogant when it comes to interview.

Substantiate your points with examples

In general, the perception of arrogance comes from the fact that the answers given lack substance. For example, saying "I would make a good doctor" could be perceived as arrogant simply because the candidate is asking the interviewer to take a statement at face value. However, if the candidate were to follow his or her initial statement with a list of the skills and attributes they possess and give examples of how they demonstrated those, then the feeling of arrogance would be removed. Substantiating your point through examples will ensure that the answer is practical and down to earth, as opposed to a vague non-proven statement.

When giving examples, focus on what you have achieved

When you give an example, it is tempting to simply list the attributes that you demonstrated but not the impact they had. Make sure you talk about the difference you made to a situation. This will give it a more concrete feel. For example, "When I talked to the old lady, I used my listening skills" sounds a little vague. However, saying "When I talked to the old lady, I spent a lot of time simply listening to her, which helped her vent her feelings and also allowed us to bond more" sounds more concrete.

If appropriate, use feedback you received from others

Saying "I have often been complimented by my teachers for being a good team player" sounds better than "I think I am a good team player".

6.3 Questions asking for examples – the STARR structure

Questions asking for examples are popular at interviews. This form of questioning, called "behavioural", stems from the fact that your recruiters are likely to learn a lot more about you by getting you to talk about your past experiences than by asking you how you might behave in hypothetical situations. Typical questions are likely to be of the form:

- Describe a situation where you worked well within a team.
- Give an example of a situation where you used your communication skills effectively.
- What is the biggest mistake you have made in the past 2 years?
- Tell us about a situation where you did not communicate well.
- When is the last time you had a conflict with someone?

Although most candidates find such questions difficult, they are in fact relatively easy once you have identified a good example to discuss, providing you follow a number of important rules.

Rule 1: Take some time to identify all the skills that you want to demonstrate

In a question such as "Describe a situation where your communication skills had a positive effect on a situation", it is obvious that the question is testing your ability to communicate but the concept of communication is still a fairly vague one. Make sure that you are clear about the specific aspects of communication that you want to emphasise. This could be:

- Your listening skills
- Your ability to relate to others through empathy
- Your ability to convey difficult issues in simple terms
- Your negotiation skills
- Your tact and diplomacy in dealing with difficult problems.

In other less obvious questions, such as "Give an example of a situation where you had to deal with a complex situation", there are many skills that you can demonstrate such as:

- Your ability to take the initiative and to work within your own limits
- Your ability to identify the resources you need to resolve this problem

- Your ability to seek help from others whenever required
- Your ability to work with your team to achieve the best possible result
- Your ability to communicate with all parties involved.

Rule 2: Make sure that you choose a specific example and that the example is relevant

When asked for an example, do not discuss vague situations or speak about your experience in general. Questions such as "Describe a situation where you played an important role in a team" often lead to answers of the type "I work in teams all the time, at school, in my summer job or at the local youth club". Giving such an answer would be missing the point of the question. If you read the question correctly, it is asking about a situation, i.e. a specific case or project that you handled. You would therefore need to be very specific.

The example also has to be relevant, i.e. it actually has to address the skill or situation asked for in the question. If you are being asked about an example of a situation where you demonstrated good communication skills, place the emphasis on how your communication skills made a difference to the outcome and not on how you were able to demonstrate leadership in resolving the problem.

Rule 3: Do not be tempted to make things up

It does not require much training to recognise a liar. Interviewers will be able to spot fairly easily whether you are making things up simply by the lack of detail that you are providing and the vagueness of your answers. And if you are caught lying, this will be very unforgiving.

Rule 4: Be personal

Describe what you did, not what everyone else did (unless it is absolutely relevant to the situation). Don't waste your time discussing what the team did and how the team worked, giving little information about what you, yourself, did. You must always remember that the point of the recruitment process is to find out about you, not about anyone else. Concentrate on the "I" rather than the "We" and don't be afraid of going into detail (provided that detail is relevant, of course).

Rule 5: Prepare examples before you go to the interview

It is notoriously difficult to come up with good examples on the spot at an interview if you have not done any preparation. Without that preparation, you will come up with examples that are lame and do not allow you to show your full potential. The range of questions asking for examples is limited and you should therefore be able to prepare adequately without wasting too much time. By preparing examples of good communication, good teamwork, leadership, initiative and creativity, a mistake that you have made, dealing with a complex situation and with a conflict situation, you will have covered 99% of the example questions normally asked.

If they are suitably complex, some of your examples can be used to illustrate different skills. For example, dealing with a difficult customer in your summer job may enable you to show good communication skills, good leadership abilities and a good aptitude for handling conflict and pressure. Preparing complex examples will therefore enable you to kill several birds with one stone and will help you minimise the number of examples that you need to remember.

Rule 6: Follow the "STARR" technique

The acronym "**STARR**" stands for:

Situation — What is the context of the story? What is the situation or project that you are discussing?

Task — What was your aim? What were you trying to achieve?

Action — What did you do? How did you go about achieving it? And why did you do it in that way?

Result — What was the end result?

Reflect — What did you feel you did well? What skills and personal attributes did you demonstrate? If relevant, what could you have done differently?

Most interviewers will have been trained in using this structure. Even if they have not, they will recognise its value when they see it. The information will be given to them in a structured manner and, as a result, they will become more receptive to the messages you are trying to communicate.

Step 1 – Situation

Describe the situation that you were confronted with or the task that needed to be accomplished. Set the context. Make it concise and informative, concentrating solely on what is useful to the story. For example, if the question is asking you to describe a situation where you had to deal with a difficult person, explain how you came to meet that person and why they were being difficult.

Step 2 – Task

Explain what you were trying to achieve. For example, if you are describing a story where your colleagues in a team were arguing about how to best handle a project, your aim might have been to encourage the team to reach a consensus without anyone being left feeling coerced or ostracised.

Step 3 – Action

This is the most important section as it is where you will need to demonstrate and highlight the skills and personal attributes that the question is testing. Now that you have set the context of your story, you need to explain what you did. In doing so, you will need to remember the following:

- Be personal, i.e. talk about you, not the rest of the team.
- Go into some detail. Do not assume that the interviewers will guess what you mean.
- Steer clear of technical information, unless it is crucial to your story.
- Explain what you did, how you did it, and why you did it.

What you did and how you did it
The interviewers will want to know how you reacted to the situation. This is where you can sell some important skills. For example, you may want to describe how you used the team to achieve a particular objective and how you kept everyone updated on progress, etc.

Why you did it

This is probably the most crucial part of your answer. Interviewers want to know that you are using a variety of generic skills in order to achieve your objectives. Therefore you must be able to demonstrate in your answer that you are taking specific actions because you are trying to achieve a specific objective and not simply by chance.

For example, when discussing a situation where you had to deal with conflict, many candidates would simply say:

I told my friend to calm down and explained to him what the problem was.

However, it would not provide a good idea of what drove you to act in this manner. How did you ask him to calm down? How did you explain the nature of the problem?

By highlighting the reasons behind your action, you would make a greater impact. For example:

I could sense that my friend was getting increasingly irritated and so, rather than argue back hoping he would understand my point, I thought it was important to allow him to talk and vent his feelings and his anger. That allowed him to calm down a little and I was then able to explain to him my own point of view on the matter, emphasising how important it was that we found a solution that suited us both.

This revised answer helps the interviewers understand what drove your actions and reinforces the feeling that you are calculating the consequences of your actions, thus retaining full control of the situation. It provides much more information about you as an individual.

Step 4 – Result

Explain what happened eventually – how it all ended. This will generally be a brief sentence designed to finish the story.

Step 5 – Reflect

So far, you have mostly been telling a story. Now is the time to tell the interviewers how this story is a good advertisement for your interpersonal skills.

For example:

Despite being confronted with a lot of resistance from my team, I was able to remain patient and confident and to constantly suggest new ways of tackling the problem. I also demonstrated a good ability to listen to others, and a good ability to stand up for my own principles.

A final statement such as this will leave a strong feeling with the interviewers and will also ensure that they are in no doubt about the points that you are trying to make through the narration of your story.

Mistakes to avoid

Questions asking for examples are some of the worst answered questions at interviews. Here are a few important points to bear in mind:

- Don't get lost in the detail of the story. Too much information will simply make it too complicated for the interviewers to understand what you are trying to convey.

- Avoid using a "theatrical" style for effect, of the type "So I said to my friend: 'Why don't we try a different approach', at which point he replied 'Well I am not sure we have time for that type of thing'. So I replied: 'It's worth trying, isn't it?'." It can be very tiring to listen to. More importantly, it forces the interviewers to focus on what was said rather than the skills and approach that you used.

- Avoid derogatory comments towards other people. For example, if you need to talk about one of your Duke of Edinburgh colleagues being too lazy, using language such as "In the end, he was being so lazy that I had to take over" will make you sound aggressive. Use neutral language such as "I felt my colleague was not as effective as the team needed him to be".

6.4 Questions relating to the role of doctors – the CAMP structure

During the course of your interview, you may be asked questions that will require some understanding of the role of doctors. This may include:

- What do you think doctors do other than treating patients?
- Where do you see yourself in 10 years' time?
- What are you hoping to achieve in your medical career?
- What challenges do you think you will face in Medicine?
- What are the pros and cons of being a doctor?

For such questions the CAMP structure can be useful:

- **C**linical   Patient care
- **A**cademic   Teaching and research
- **M**anagement   Managing others, running & developing services
- **P**ersonal   Personal attributes, hobbies

Here is an example of how CAMP can be used:

Q: What do you think doctors do other than treating patients?

- **Clinical**   They have meetings to discuss complex cases and they invest time in keeping up to date, e.g. by reading journals, attending courses, etc.

- **Academic**   They teach medical students, trainees and other professionals. They also undertake research.

- **Management** They manage and support other colleagues, get involved in patient safety, quality improvement and service development projects.

- **Personal**   They try to have a life as well.

6.5 Expressing an opinion

Questions asking for your opinion are not designed to test whether your ideas match those of the panel. Indeed, you are allowed to think what you want, provided you can justify your opinions with sensible arguments and avoid coming across as bigoted. Instead, what the panel will require from you is an ability to think about a given topic from different perspectives, to present balanced arguments in a clear, concise and structured manner and to discuss issues in an adult fashion with them.

When asked for an opinion, you should ensure that you present arguments on both sides of the debate before giving your own opinion.

In most cases, the opinions that you are required to give are related to topics which are either in the news at the time of the interview (new research, court case), an ongoing political issue (role of nurses, NHS reforms) or an ethical issue or scenario (abortion, euthanasia, vivisection, liver transplants for alcoholics, etc.). In some cases, such as ethical dilemmas, it may prove impossible to give a definite opinion; however, whenever possible I would suggest that you do not sit too much on the fence and that you provide a definite answer.

Here are a few examples (note that we have simplified the answers in order to illustrate the technique to answer the question rather than provide a full list of arguments to answer each question):

Was it a good idea to send a man to the moon?

There are many reasons why this was a good idea. For example, it made a huge contribution to the advancement of science, and in many ways it also contributed to boost the morale of the nations involved with it. However, on the flipside, it did cost a huge amount of money, which could have been used towards other more worthwhile causes such as <name a few causes that you value>, though that would probably only have had a temporary effect. So on balance I would say that it was a good idea because I feel the positives outweigh the negatives.

Note how, in this example, the candidate has given arguments for and against before formulating their own opinion.

Do you think doctors should ever go on strike?

There is certainly a case for doctors to be allowed to strike. That could particularly be the case when they want to highlight issues relating to patient safety to the government and the general public. However, this can also be counterproductive as doctors are generally considered to be well-off and most of the general population may not fully comprehend why doctors feel the need to strike over issues such as pay and pensions. So overall, the answer is yes provided doctors fight the right battles.

Here again, the candidate presents both sides of the argument before concluding.

Do you think it is right for carers to encourage relatives to go to Switzerland for euthanasia?

Euthanasia is a sensitive topic. There are situations where it could be argued that the quality of life of a patient has deteriorated so much that their dying may become a welcome solution to their suffering. On the other hand, it is difficult to argue that human beings should have the right of life and death on one another; or that a carer is best placed to make decisions on behalf of a relative who may not be fully able to express their own wishes.

Overall, I am not sure whether I agree with it or not. In fact, there are days where I agree and others where I disagree. I guess that is why decisions such as these are left to each individual to mull over for themselves, and why the decision to prosecute individuals is handled by the authorities on a case-by-case basis.

In this answer the candidate has not expressed an opinion either way, but has shown that he/she is able to find arguments for and against. An alternative conclusion could have been:

From a religious perspective, I am firmly against the idea that we should interfere with the life of another human being in such a way as to terminate their life. However, I can see why some people may think differently and they are entitled to their own thoughts on the topic.

This conclusion is that of a candidate with firm convictions. There is nothing wrong with having convictions, religious or otherwise, provided you can demonstrate an understanding that others may feel differently so as not to appear judgemental.

Preparing for questions asking for opinions

In order to deal with current issues or political issues, you will need to be familiar with the details and this book will help you a lot in understanding some of the intricacies. However, you would be well advised to spend some time reading relevant news websites and newspapers as they are often a rich source of arguments that you can use in your own answers.

In order to deal with ethical issues, you will also need to have done a substantial amount of thinking and reading in your own time so that you can acquire a good ability to debate. This book will give you many arguments that you can use. However, to complement it, you will need to spend some time discussing them informally with friends and family. You will be all the more equipped for having listened to and argued with your closest friends or relatives. The interviewers will expect you to engage in a similar debate with them.

6.6 Dealing with confrontational interviewers

Some interviewers will be keen to test whether you can deal well with pressure; and whether you have thought your arguments out or are simply regurgitating something you have learnt. A common way in which they might achieve all those objectives is by deliberately arguing with some of the points you have just made. This may lead to exchanges of the type:

You:
I feel that being a doctor will help me make a different to people's lives.

Interviewer:
Do you really think we make a real difference?

Or

You:
I feel that Manchester is one of the best medical schools because ...

Interviewer:
You applied to three other medical schools. I bet you are saying that to everyone.

You:
Well yes, obviously; most people have. For example I applied to Barts too but I think that Manchester would be better because ...

Interviewer:
I trained at Barts. Are you saying my training was inferior?

Or

You:
To choose who can get a liver transplant I would need to assess a number of parameters before a decision could be made.

Interviewer:
So basically you are sitting on the fence.

Although such situations are not uncommon, your first reaction should be to be flattered. If they argue with you, in general that means that they care. If they found you beyond repair, they will often just move on.

Your second reaction should be to stop and ask yourself why they are acting in that way. Here is a mini guide on how to handle the different scenarios:

Scenario 1: You have said something wrong on a factual question

If you said something which, with hindsight, you realise is wrong, simply apologise for your mistake, tell them that they are correct and then move on. They will appreciate your honesty and integrity. If you persist in arguing that you were right anyway, or if you try to diminish your mistake by pretending you were kind of right, then you will score very low.

Scenario 2: They are querying something that you think is correct

Don't be afraid to stand up for yourself but make sure that you back up what you say in the nicest possible way. They might just be testing that you actually meant what you said. For example:

Interviewer:
Do you really think that doctors make a real difference?

You:
Yes I do. There are many situations I can think of where doctors really make a difference. For example, <give examples>.

I am sure that, as you suggest, there are cases where it can appear that we make little difference. For example, I have seen during my GP work experience that some patients can be so stubborn that it is hard to see what more one can do for them. But, even in such cases, one can argue that, by keeping them engaged and by communicating with them, we are keeping the lines of communication open; and in the end this may well pay off.

Scenario 3: They are querying something where there is no definite answer

Such situations can rapidly degenerate into a real ping-pong match. For example:

You:
Doctors should not strike, because it destroys the trust patients have in them.

Interviewer:
In the end patients have to come to you anyway, so what difference does that make?

You:
Perhaps but doctors also owe patients respect and there would really need to be a good reason for them to strike.

Interviewer:
Do you not think that pensions and pay are a good enough reason?

If you continue this conversation, you will see more and more topics being drawn into it, with no real chance of finding a mutually satisfactory answer to the original problem. In fact, you might even risk losing your patience, or worse, your temper.

A good way of handling such situations is to stop the conversation and to go back to first principles very quickly. For example:

I think that, at the end of the day, I am sure we can find multiple arguments for and against and that all are valid in their own way. It is also a very subjective issue so everyone is entitled to have a different opinion. I think that, fundamentally, what we are trying to achieve is to ensure that doctors have the means to defend themselves, but at the same time that patient safety is not compromised.

Don't worry if you can't find a definite answer. There isn't always one.

7 Questions on motivation & interest in medical issues

7.1 Why do you want to study Medicine?

Many candidates launch straight into an explanation without having first clarified in their own mind why they actually want to be a doctor. To give a good answer, you must analyse those reasons and recollect the process that you followed to identify Medicine as a career.

There are many reasons why people want to study Medicine. These may include:

- A strong interest in science
- Wanting to go into a challenging profession
- Wanting to help others
- Wanting a profession that combines intellectual abilities and a strong element of communication
- Being interested by the variety of work involved, from prevention to treatment but also teaching, research, etc.
- Enjoying close contact with people, and making a difference to their lives
- Wanting to work in an environment where there is a strong element of teamwork
- Enjoying constant learning.

All these reasons are laudable and you must ensure that your own reasons are clear in your mind. The main problem at interviews is that the reasons above are likely to be mentioned by most people. If you simply list a few of them then your answer will be bland and will resemble 700 other answers.

However, this does not mean that the above facts must be rejected. They are an important aspect of the answer and should be addressed too.

How can you stand out?

Firstly, it is important to realise that sounding different does not necessarily mean that you have to find a reason that no one else has thought about. In other words, you don't need to present an obscure reason for choosing Medicine in order to sound interesting. Instead, you should identify your true reasons and develop them well.

Secondly, you must make your answer personal and deliver it in an enthusiastic style. Repeating five times in your answer that you are really keen on Medicine will not make your point any stronger. Your enthusiasm will come across through the way you speak and the personal nature of your answers. The following should help you out:

1. **Choose three or four reasons only**
    It is better to concentrate on a handful of points that you develop well, than to develop 25 different ideas in 2 seconds each. In other words quality is better than quantity.

2. **Explain each reason clearly**
    Many will say that they enjoy science, but it is hardly a convincing argument by itself. It is also quite difficult to convey your enthusiasm for science through such a simple statement. Instead, try to back this statement up by explaining what you enjoy about science. Is it the intellectual challenge of having to use facts and judgement to resolve problems (in which case you will enjoy diagnosing patients)? Is it the fact that it is both intellectual and practical (in which case, Medicine is definitely a good field to get into)?

    Similarly, it is easy to state that Medicine is challenging. However, an interviewer might find your answer more interesting if you explain why you feel that it will challenge you. Is it the fact that you will have to deal with the unexpected? Or maybe the fact that it is a constant learning curve, that you have to keep up to date and that it involves working with many people with different skills and personalities? Whatever the reason, you need to develop it so that the interviewers are not fed quick headlines but a really personal point of view.

3. **Use your work experience and other personal experiences**
   In many cases, the reasons that you chose Medicine as a career will have been highlighted through the personal experience that you have gained of Medicine. In your work experience, you might have seen first hand how medical teams work; you might have had personal experience of the impact of good listening and empathy on particular patients, or had exposure to the wonders of technology.

   Everything counts and helps in making your answer stand out. To make it personal you will need to go into some detail about what you have seen and experienced, and, more importantly, how this has made you feel and how these experiences have reinforced your career choice.

Example of an effective answer

Medicine is a career that I have had in mind for a very long time and which I have learnt to appreciate even more over the past year during my work experience.

I have always been very interested in science, whether this was biology or physics, and I have a very inquisitive mind. I have always been fascinated by the complexities of the human body, the intricate mix of the biological and the chemical and also the manner in which the human psyche can interact with the physical. Over the past few years I have read up on many medical and scientific issues. For example, I read quite a lot about the measles epidemic in Wales when it broke out and at the moment I am following closely the current debate on euthanasia. I feel that going into Medicine will really give me a good opportunity to work in an intellectually challenging environment.

I really enjoy taking care of others. I have been a volunteer for St John Ambulance since the age of 15 and I have spent a lot of time providing first aid at major events. I also recently spent some time working for a helpline for suicidal people. These two experiences have really helped me to understand more about the various pains that people can experience, from the physical to the psychological. I enjoyed both experiences because I could feel that I was making a real difference to those people, if only by offering a reassuring presence. This reinforced in me the desire to get into a profession where I would make a difference at a personal level and that Medicine was really the path that I wanted to follow.

As well as all this, I am greatly interested by the vast opportunities and the variety that Medicine offers. As part of my work experience, I had the opportunity to shadow a consultant anaesthetist who shared his time between clinical work and research. This gave me a good insight into the numerous roles that doctors play. As well as managing the care of his patients, he spent time supervising and teaching junior colleagues or carrying out his research. I also had the opportunity to shadow a GP for 3 weeks, and gained a first-hand understanding of how the doctors are not just clinicians but they are also educators and counsellors. I find this range of activities very exciting.

Overall, I feel that Medicine offers everything that I am looking for in a career: an intellectual challenge, an environment where teamwork and communication play an important part, a close proximity to people, and, more than any other profession, a true feeling of being able to make a real difference to my surrounding environment.

This answer is on the long side but it develops well each of the arguments brought forward by the candidate. Note how it is made up of three paragraphs (not too many points) framed by an introduction and a conclusion. Each paragraph starts with a message, which is then backed up by experience in the text. This provides a clear structure that enables the listener to keep track of the main reasons being highlighted.

In the example above, each point is backed up by two experiences. If your speed of delivery is slow or if you feel uncomfortable with answers on the longer side, then the answer could be made shorter by simply mentioning one experience in each paragraph instead. Whether you take a short or a long approach, make sure your answer fits within a 1.5- to 3-minute window. They need to have time to ask you other questions too!

Do you need to have had an early interest in Medicine?

A good way of introducing your answer to the "Why Medicine?" questions is to talk about how your interest in Medicine started. For example, some candidates have had serious conditions themselves and through these they have been exposed substantially to the medical profession, which has prompted their interest. Some may have nursed elderly relatives throughout their youth and discovered their vocation in this way; others may have had experience of voluntary work with disadvantaged people, whether in the UK or abroad, and developed an interest in "making a difference" from an early age.

If you have been in such a situation, you may find that it is useful to use it to fully personalise your answer. However, most people have not been exposed to such circumstances and, in an effort to be personal, they tend to provide answers with a forced personalisation that could sound corny, such as:

▪ "I broke my leg when I was ten and I was fascinated by the work that doctors did on it. This really made me want to be a doctor."

   Maybe so, but it runs the risk of sounding a little weak. It is a bit like saying "My sister does jigsaw puzzles and I really want to do this for a living." We are all exposed to different events in our lives and we are obviously influenced by all of them. However, these days, you see more medical drama on TV than you would see at the hospital when breaking a leg and the jump from the broken leg to a medical vocation is slightly weak.

▪ "I used to visit my Nan at the hospital and found it fascinating to see how the nurses cared for her."

   Again, we all observe events in our lives and you would need to have been strongly influenced and to have been marked sufficiently by that situation to justify its link to your career in Medicine. Many people find the work of firemen fascinating but have never really thought of making a career of it. Observing a situation does not mean that you would be good at working within that setting unless you could demonstrate the extent of your feelings following your exposure. In this example, you would get more mileage out of explaining what you gained from caring for your Nan and helping her through her illness from a physical and psychological point of view than by observing how others cared for her.

There is no real harm in mentioning personal events, but you should make sure that you don't give them an importance that they don't necessarily deserve in reality.

Should you say that there are doctors in your family?

A number of applicants have taken the medical route because someone in their family is a doctor and they have gained exposure to the system from an early age. In principle, there is nothing wrong with mentioning it, although you should realise that this will not be sufficient to get you a place. Interviewers will be more concerned about whether you have what it takes rather than whether you were born into the right family. Therefore you should identify in your experience the elements that made you grow as a person and you should avoid dwelling too much on what you have observed or heard from others in your family. The last thing you want is to give the impression that you are only there because your family thought it might be a good idea. Generally speaking, you should be able to put forward a convincing argument without mentioning that your family is full of doctors.

Conclusion: if you can avoid it, then avoid it. At the very least, keep your references to the bare minimum. You will get more credit by talking about the work experience that you have organised by yourself and from which you have personally gained than from a ready-made experience handed to you by relatives. You must show drive and initiative as well as personal will.

What if you are a young graduate?

There are two main types of graduates: those who have already tried to enter medical school before and those who have not.

If you have already attempted medical school before then you should explain how the past few years have helped you to mature in your decision to become a doctor. As part of that process, you should also address the additional skills that you gained during your degree.

If you have never attempted medical school before, then you will need to explain how the past few years have made a difference. In some cases, it pays to be honest by explaining what your original career intentions were and by setting out how you discovered your vocation for Medicine.

What if you are a mature applicant?

A number of candidates go into medical school at a later stage in life. Such candidates are welcome because they bring a range of attributes and maturity that is not always found in younger students. They usually show more motivation as their decision to join Medicine tends to be deliberate rather than impulsive. In many ways, this should make it easier to explain your motivation towards Medicine because you will have followed a personal journey to reach that decision and therefore should have more arguments than most to explain your new-found vocation.

The only real approach that you can take is to explain how you came to choose your first career and to detail the process through which you changed your mind. There are a number of factors that you should bear in mind:

- **Never be ashamed of your past and never present the situation in an apologetic manner.** No one has a straightforward life and people from very different backgrounds can be good doctors regardless of how they got there.

- **Never criticise your old career.** You do not want to give the impression that you are choosing an alternative career as a knee-jerk reaction. It is likely that there are aspects of your old career that you will have found less satisfactory than others, but you should try to present these in the context of all the good aspects of that job and the learning and maturity that you have drawn from it.

- **Highlight the similarities between your old career and Medicine** and explain why you feel Medicine will add an extra dimension. So for example:

    - Someone who worked in a legal practice before will have enjoyed the client facing aspect, the opportunity to make a difference to people's lives and to work in an intellectually challenging environment, but might be frustrated at the fact that a lot of the work is paperwork as opposed to practical.

    - Someone who worked in engineering might have enjoyed its scientific side, the research side and the fact that they could make a difference to how the world works, but might be frustrated at the lack of direct human contact with those whose lives are affected.

    - Someone who worked in politics might have enjoyed the opportunity to get involved in society and make a difference but might be frustrated by the lack of direct action (too much talking!).

7.2 Why not nursing or another healthcare profession?

This question is often interpreted as a trap when it is merely testing your motivation in greater depth. Do not take such open questioning as a sign that your first answer was not appropriate. Instead, use this as an opportunity to demonstrate your understanding of the roles played by doctors, nurses and other professionals, and how they complement one another.

Beware of the common traps

- "Doctors can prescribe" – True, but so can some nurses, albeit under certain conditions.

- "Doctors can make decisions" – Are you saying nurses can't?

- "Being a doctor is more interesting" – Go and say that to a nurse!

- "Doctors can make a real difference to patients; nurses merely follow orders." Doctors often find that nurses can achieve much more than they themselves can simply because nurses spend more time with patients and are often better able to communicate and empathise. Though it is true that many aspects of nursing are controlled by protocol, it does not mean they make less of a difference.

- "There are better career prospects for doctors." Given the fact that there are areas where there are 1000 applicants for one post, this is not a very clever argument. In any case, some nurses can develop high flying careers too, for example as nurse practitioners or nurse consultants. In some cases, they may even earn more than doctors.

How to approach the question

1. Do not criticise nurses. You will have to work with them and there may even be some on the panel. The main problem with the arguments above is that they are too simplistic.

2. You can give similar arguments to those described above, but you will need to be more explicit. You should also illustrate your arguments with examples. Arguments that may be used include:

i. Doctors receive a general training, which ensures that they have knowledge and experience of clinical areas beyond their specialty. This aids the management of the patient when matters beyond that specialty are important.

ii. Doctors have ultimate responsibility for the patient. They are driving the decision-making process. Although nurses contribute greatly to that process, the final decision will rest with a doctor.

iii. Both nurses and doctors may get involved in research activities. However, doctors are more likely to take a lead in the research projects while nurses may be more involved in the actual practical execution of projects.

iv. Although nurse practitioners undergo similar training to medical students, for clinical examination, for instance, they do not meet the standards of clinical skills that doctors are able to achieve after taking postgraduate examinations (e.g. exams for membership of Royal Colleges).

v. It is true that, nowadays, some nurses have taken roles traditionally taken by doctors, particularly in the domains of investigation, diagnosis and treatment, and that the gap has narrowed. But:

- Only a small minority have the opportunity to become involved in these activities, and only in very specialised areas. The activities of these nurses are highly protocol driven, leaving little leeway for discretion (i.e. basically the art of Medicine);

- Nurse specialists have clinical expertise in that specialty only, whereas the doctors, due to their medical training, will have knowledge and experience of clinical areas beyond that specialty. For example, a TB specialist nurse managing a patient with a history of liver problems may run into problems when considering anti-tuberculosis treatment and will require the involvement of a specialist doctor.

3. Make sure that you praise the role of nurses and mention how important they are to the care of patients. Emphasise that it is not a matter of one being better than the other but of people with different levels of responsibility and skills working together towards one goal.

Why not any other healthcare profession?

Your answer to this should start with "Indeed, why not?" Many healthcare professions have a lot in common with the role of doctors (close contact with patient, caring patient-centred approach, etc.) and in many respects they are joined by people who have similar personal characteristics to those exhibited by doctors.

In the first instance, you should highlight the similarities between other healthcare professions and being a doctor, thereby showing your understanding that it is not as simple as "them and us". You can then follow this with a highlight of some of the differences. These would include the differences highlighted above between nurses and doctors, as well as the fact that doctors can prescribe and diagnose, which adds to the challenge.

7.3 What steps have you taken to find out whether Medicine is the right career for you?

This question is designed to test two things:

1. Drive and initiative – to demonstrate this, you will need to talk about the various steps that you have taken to test your interest in the medical profession.

2. Enthusiasm and determination – to demonstrate this, you will need to talk about your experiences from a personal point of view, highlighting not only what you did and observed but also introducing an element of personal reflection by discussing what you enjoyed about these experiences and how they contributed to reinforcing your vocation.

The various "steps" you can mention

Obviously, during the period leading to your decision to apply for Medicine, you will have undertaken a range of activities that will have given you an understanding of the role and responsibilities of doctors. The following list should prompt your memory (or give you some ideas if you are planning to gain some experience in the forthcoming months):

- Attending seminars (e.g. introduction to a life in Medicine)
- Attending open days at a local hospital and at any medical school
- Discussing your aspirations with a doctor
- Work experience in a local hospital or shadowing a nurse or a GP
- Working as a healthcare assistant or a hospital porter
- Working with disabled children or in a hospice
- Working as a temporary medical secretary.

All these give you an opportunity to learn about Medicine in different ways:

- Seminars and open days can give you a chance to discuss your aspirations with people who work in the field and are therefore very informative.

- Work experience is a good opportunity to see Medicine from the inside and to understand what being a doctor is about. It also gives you opportunities to experience patient contact.

How to approach the question

The list of possible work experiences is limited and most candidates will have made some kind of effort to test their vocation. In order to stand out, you will need to produce an answer that presents your own experience in an interesting manner rather than simply listing the two or three hospitals in which you worked.

In practice, this means detailing each experience, how you organised it and, most importantly, what you learnt from it and how it contributed to your decision to get into Medicine.

Example of an ineffective answer

I went to a couple of seminars and also shadowed a doctor for 2 weeks during the summer break. It was really interesting and it really made me realise that I wanted to do Medicine.

What is wrong with it?

- It lacks detail. What kind of seminars? What kind of doctor did he shadow? What did he observe? And how did he organise the shadowing (the candidate may have missed an opportunity to sell his personal initiative)?

- There is no personal reflection. The candidate should have expanded on some of his key messages: what was interesting and why? How did the experience make him realise that Medicine was a career that he would enjoy?

Generally speaking, you should avoid using words such as "interesting", "fascinating", "enlightening", "excellent", etc. by themselves. Whenever you use one of these words or other words designed to express personal feelings, explain why you felt that way.

7.4 What have you read or experienced to prepare for entry into Medicine?

This question is very similar to Q.7.3: "What steps have you taken to find out whether Medicine is the right career for you?" and you may choose to use a similar answer. Since the question asks explicitly what you have read or experienced, you will need to address both aspects. You could divide your answer between essential and desirable preparation.

Essential preparation
- A Level subjects such as biochemistry, biology and mathematics
- Saw career advisers and enquired about the various medical schools
- Read the medical schools' prospectuses
- Visited the medical schools (open days or by yourself)
- Spoke to the medical students
- Organised work experience in GP practice, hospital or hospice.

Desirable preparation
- Attended introductory course or seminar for Medicine
- Read relevant medical journals (*Lancet*, *BMJ*, etc.)
- Read articles from the *studentBMJ* or other magazine/paper
- Read about healthcare issues, such as postcode lottery, in national newspaper on websites, newspapers or other media
- Read and researched ethical issues posed by current court cases
- Worked for charities such as Oxfam and Hospice
- Summer jobs in a hospital such as porter or healthcare assistant.

Summarise the extent of your experience. Select the main activities that you have undertaken and describe what you did and observed there. Ensure that you bring an element of personal reflection on each activity, describing why you enjoyed each experience and how this made you understand Medicine and/or the role of doctors. When talking about what you have read, explain what you learnt from it and why it made an interesting read.

Example of an effective answer

One of my first steps was to arrange a meeting with my school careers adviser, following which I arranged to shadow a consultant anaesthetist at my local hospital. I spent 2 weeks observing the consultant both in his clinics and in theatre. It was very exciting to see a patient being given general anaesthesia before undertaking a major ENT operation. It really gave me a good insight into the different roles played by doctors, ranging from communicating with the patient before the operation to obtain consent and to reassure them about the procedure, all the way to actually carrying out the anaesthesia and the clinical knowledge and judgement that this requires. I also found the teamwork aspect of the job very inspiring, particularly the fact that the team was very well coordinated and worked well together to benefit the patient. From a personal point of view, I had the opportunity to have a chat with the patients that we managed both before and after their operation and I could see the impact that our discussions had on them, if only as a means of reassurance.

I have also worked with disabled children for a local charity, helping them with their homework and helping the carers during day trips. It was hard work and could sometimes be disheartening, but I have always found it very rewarding. It really taught me the importance of being patient with the children and to involve them as much as possible in resolving the issues that they faced. Although it was evident from the beginning that not all these children would manage by themselves, it was really rewarding to see the progress that they all made, however little this was.

Overall, I feel that my work experience has been really useful and has really reaffirmed in me the fact that Medicine is a career that I will thrive in and through which I will most benefit others.

Note the depth added by having two experiences of a different nature (one geared towards observation and one geared towards personal experience) and the manner in which personal feelings are described and explained, which helps make the answer personal and interesting to an interviewer's ear. The simple two-point structure contributes greatly to the clarity of the answer.

7.5 Tell us about your work experience

This question is also similar in nature to Q.7.3: "What steps have you taken to find out whether Medicine is the right career for you?" and the approach to answering it should be nearly identical, the only difference being that the question is asking you to concentrate on work experience rather than any other activities such as attending relevant seminars or open days.

Do not make assumptions about how much the interviewers know and how much they might have read or not read about you

Interviewers will normally have read your personal statement, either at shortlisting stage and/or just before the interview itself. However, they will also have read personal statements from many other candidates and may therefore need you to refresh their memory. It is your job to make sure that they get the right message. That means banning phrases such as "As you have seen in my personal statement" or "As you know". Build a personal answer from scratch.

Be descriptive and personal

Refer to the answer to Q.7.3. for a full explanation of how to approach this type of question. In your answer you need to describe the extent of your experience: if possible, how you organised the work experience, what you observed and what you gained from a personal point of view. Explain what you enjoyed and, most importantly, why you enjoyed it and how it helped you decide in favour of a medical career.

Example of an ineffective answer

Last year, I shadowed an anaesthetist and an A&E consultant, which I enjoyed tremendously. I also did my summer job at my local hospital as a healthcare assistant and now I know what it is like to work in a hospital. I have also done some work experience at the local GP practice.

What is wrong with it?

- Good mix of experience but we don't know whether the candidate was just making cups of tea and watching TV during that time, or whether he actually learnt a lot from these experiences
- "I know what it is like to work in a hospital." What is it like?
- No details and no reflection on each of these experiences
- Knowing what it is like to work in a hospital does not mean that he liked it. How did this experience contribute to reinforce Medicine as a career for him?

Example of an effective answer

I have done work experience both at my local hospital and my local GP practice and I found that it really helped me in identifying and thinking about the challenges that I will face as a doctor.

At the hospital, I observed a busy team in the oncology department, which showed me the practical side of dealing with patient care. One of my main learning points has been that being a doctor is a lot of hard work, which I feel I am prepared to take on, but that it can also be very rewarding. The team had a number of good successes with some of their patients and the efforts that the team put in really paid off. During my time there, I had the opportunity to attend some team meetings as well as some multidisciplinary meetings. Through this, I gained a good insight into how doctors and other health professionals pull their expertise together for the good of patients and I found this particularly enriching. I also gained a lot from my personal experience in dealing with patients and, through this, about the importance for doctors to be skilled in many areas and not just in terms of clinical skills.

When I worked in the community at the local GP surgery, I observed the holistic approach of the GP. I have learnt the importance of good communication and demonstrating empathy. I particularly liked the way patients are treated for all their physical, psychological and social needs.

I feel that I have learnt a lot from my work experience and I am looking forward to starting Medicine as soon as possible so that I can continue to experience the feelings and the buzz that I experienced during these assignments.

7.6 Tell us about your gap year

This question is similar to previous questions about work experience or how you prepared for a career in Medicine. Its main purpose is to test not only your determination to enter a career in Medicine by looking at the medical experience that you gained during that year, but also your organisational skills and initiative by looking at how you went about organising your gap year.

There is no harm in discussing time taken off for a holiday providing it did not last the entire year, but this will need to be done in an appropriate manner, i.e. always trying to emphasise personal learning or selling personal attributes such as initiative and organisation skills.

Similarly to the questions discussed previously, the recipe for a good answer lies in the following:

- A good mix of experience, with a brief description of what it entailed
- Drawing attention to what you gained from that experience rather than simply describing how interesting it was
- Emphasising how this helped you towards a career in Medicine.

Example of an effective answer

My gap year was a valuable experience in many respects. I travelled with my friends to South America in the first 2 months after the exams. This gave me a good opportunity to relax and condition myself for the rest of the year. I really enjoyed preparing for the trip, having to plan our itinerary, finding suitable accommodation and working to save money so that we could afford it. Once there, it was good to experience a different culture and we saw some really fantastic places.

I then spent 6 months working with disabled children in Chile. I found the experience very humbling and enriching from a personal point of view. I learnt a lot from working there and, in particular, how important teamwork is when you have to deal with both day-to-day and complex issues. Because we had few resources, we needed to use whatever resources were available and to use one another's skills to succeed in helping the children out. It also really taught me that, when all else fails, communication is very important. Although we knew that some of the children would never really have a very good life, it was amazing to see what difference we could make simply by listening to them and showing generosity and empathy.

After a fantastic 6 months I came back home to work as a healthcare assistant at my local hospital in Colchester. As well as helping me out financially to repay the loan I had taken out to finance the trip to South America, it gave me an excellent opportunity to work in a UK medical environment. During that time, I had many opportunities to have close patient contact and to observe how doctors and nurses work closely together in a very busy environment.

During my gap year, I learnt an awful lot from a personal perspective. In particular, I feel that I have leant to be more mature, responsible and organised. It has really reinforced in me the desire to become a doctor.

If your gap year is not yet over at the time of the interview then you should also talk about the projects that you have for the remainder of the year, emphasising what you are hoping to get out of it.

7.7 What would you do if you were unsuccessful at getting into Medicine this year?

The answer to this question will depend on your current situation. The point here is that you should demonstrate drive and motivation to become a doctor while being realistic.

If you are applying for the first time

In this situation you have no choice but to give the message that you will be trying again. Giving up at the first opportunity would be interpreted as a serious lack of motivation. It is most important that you appear as someone who is motivated and energetic and your answer should also discuss the steps that you would take to gain further experience and maturity while you are waiting to reapply. In most cases, this would consist of a productive gap year. When you describe your planned activities ensure that they bear some relation to Medicine (you would get severely penalised for saying that you want to go wind-surfing for a year). An example of good answer would be:

I have had a passion for Medicine since a young age and I am determined to do everything possible to gain entry to medical school. If I do not get into a medical school this year, I will of course be very disappointed but I know that I will also be able to rely on support from my friends and family. My first step will be to identify the weaknesses in my CV and in my interview skills by getting feedback from the medical school and other people I can trust. This will help me improve my application for next time.

I will also organise a gap year. During that time I intend to get involved in healthcare work experience and charity work, such as working for the Red Cross and St John Ambulance. I would also like to shadow doctors at my local hospital for some time in order to familiarise myself further with the medical profession and possibly to get involved in working in a scientific lab to find out more about medical research.

I would also like to take some time out to go travelling before applying again for medical school next year. I am particularly interested in South America and I may be able to organise a long trip to Chile where I would be able to combine a holiday with an involvement in local charity work.

If you are a re-applicant totally focused on Medicine

If this is not your first application then you will need to provide a realistic view of the situation. There is little point in mentioning that you will keep trying until you reach the age of 65.

We have seen cases of candidates applying six times in a row, who thought that applying again and again showed that they were motivated. That may be the case for the second or third attempt but there comes a time where you have to show common sense and show an understanding that enough is enough and that you simply cannot put your life on hold for a distant ambition.

In most cases, you will be able to do a degree that will enable you to get back to Medicine at a later stage. Do not forget that the answer to this question should sell your motivation, and not simply admit defeat. For example:

Although I am passionate and determined to pursue a career in Medicine, I understand that this is my third consecutive year in applying for medical school.

This year, I have tried my absolute best to enhance my CV in terms of academic achievements, generic skills and experience in the medical field. In particular, I have gained a lot of maturity through my work experience. I really hope this will demonstrate my strength and dedication in a medical career.

However, if I fail to get in again, I will apply for a pharmacy degree. I am confident that by practising pharmacy both in a hospital and in the community and by getting exposed to patients on a daily basis, I will have a job that I enjoy. As well as giving me some useful skills and knowledge, this degree will enable me to re-apply to Medicine as a postgraduate or mature student entrant later on.

Obviously, any degree relevant to healthcare would be equally suitable, ranging from biochemistry and biology to pharmacy or even dentistry (whose students often have common lectures with medical students).

If you are a re-applicant but have seriously thought about an alternative career

Many people will mention the fact that, should they fail, they will do a related degree and will try again in a few years' time. This is a good strategy, but with a small risk that the interviewers will have heard it all before. You may also be at a stage where you have already done the degree and another degree is not an option. Remember that the point of this question is to test your aptitude for Medicine and therefore your personal attributes. There are other careers that may look very different to Medicine but in fact have many similarities.

For example, law is a career where you will have contact with people, where you will need to build a strong rapport with your clients, understand issues from their point of view, study a great deal and make use of your knowledge and best judgement to make important decisions (not dissimilar to the art of diagnosing). So, mentioning that you have thought about a career in law would not be a totally absurd idea, providing it is well presented. Other possible alternatives include social services, psychology or generally any professions that are centred on improving quality of life.

This can be a risky strategy but may reap greater rewards if you have the personality to pull it off.

7.8 Where do you see yourself in 10 years' time?

This question is a mystery to most candidates since what they will be doing is fairly obvious: *"I will be a doctor of course, but I am not sure what kind yet."* Such an answer reveals very little about the candidate him/herself and therefore it is unlikely to have any kind of impact at an interview.

Not mentioning the fact that it is almost telling the interviewers that they have asked a stupid question, which can't help much.

Example of an ineffective answer

I see myself being a final year medical student finishing my medical training in 5 years' time and becoming a doctor in a busy teaching hospital treating sick patients in 10 years' time. I hope I can achieve these goals.

As well as stating the obvious in several places, the answer does not provide any information that would help the interviewers grasp the candidate's motivation. Also, the end is not very encouraging. One would think that a candidate would more than "hope" and would instead take control of the situation to maximise their chances of success.

How to approach the question

This question offers a perfect opportunity to outline the objectives you set for yourself using the CAMP framework (see Section 6.4), which will enable you to address your ambitions from different perspectives: clinical, academic, management and personal.

A good answer will show that you have an interest in developing yourself in a multidimensional fashion and that you have some sense of direction. By using the CAMP framework, you will also show a good understanding of the different aspects of life as a doctor (see also Q.7.15: "What do doctors do apart from treating patients?" for ideas).

Example of an effective answer

Medical school will have given me a good background and a solid base on which to build a career as a doctor. During my work experience, I have really enjoyed my time shadowing a surgeon at my local hospital and I think I would really enjoy taking up a specialty which has a strong practical dimension; though, obviously, my medical training over the next 5 years may open my eyes to other opportunities.

From an academic perspective, I am very interested in teaching. I have already built some good teaching experience by mentoring two children at my local school and by being a football coach on Wednesday evenings over the past 2 years. It is something that I enjoy very much and I would like to think that teaching others will form a central part of my future job as a doctor. Also, though I don't have any experience of research so far, I have read many articles based on clinical research and this is an activity in which I would like to get involved at some stage.

As you will have seen from my personal statement, I am someone who enjoys taking responsibility. I am particularly proud of what I achieved as marketing manager within the Young Enterprise project, and I would cer-tainly like to continue taking responsibilities when I graduate. During my work experience I had the opportunity to sit on some of the meetings at-tended by the consultant and saw that there are many opportunities for doctors to be involved in managerial activities and I think that this would suit me well. Part of what attracts me to Medicine is in fact the variety of roles and so I would like to think that I can contribute to Medicine in more than one way.

Finally, I am a keen cyclist in my spare time and would like to think that I will still have some time to pursue this as a hobby. I would also like to start a family once my career path is more settled.

Note the attempt to personalise the answer by bringing past experiences of teaching and hobbies into it.

7.9 If you had the choice between being a GP, a surgeon or a physician, which would you choose?

At first, it is tempting to sit on the fence and, in an effort to upset no one and to give a "one-size-fits-all" answer, to simply answer that you have no idea at this stage and that you will use your time at medical school to find out about the different specialties before you can make a choice. In reality, you should bear in mind a number of important facts:

- The vast majority of candidates will give the answer written above. Giving the same one may seem like playing it safe but you are not really adding value or trying to stand out. Without being definite about your career choice, you can still find a way to sound a bit more determined and aware of the different medical careers that suit you.

- If you have already made your choice, it is okay to show that you have a good idea of what you want to do. It shows that you have thought about your career and it will make you appear more motivated than the "sitting-on-the-fence" candidates. However, since your experience of the medical environment is fairly limited at this stage, you should ensure that you remain open-minded, at least for the sake of the interview. In particular, you do not want to give the impression that you will study your preferred specialty at medical school and that you will neglect the rest.

- GPs, surgeons and physicians tend to have personalities that are adapted to the type of work that they do ("tend to" because, of course, there are plenty of exceptions). Your personality may be more adapted to one or two of these three choices.

- You will not get better marked for choosing one option or another. The key in this question is your motivation and the reasoning behind your answer.

The facts

To help you, we have summarised below some of the more commonly accepted work- and personality-related characteristics of each of these three career choices.

General Practitioner (GP)
- Holistic approach to patient care (i.e. looking after not only the clinical aspect but also the psychological and social aspects)
- Continuity of care – GPs can follow their patients from "cradle to grave" and deal with all aspects of their care. Effectively GPs can be seen as Health Managers
- Work in the community rather than in a hospital
- Enjoy variety in their work including:
    - Dealing with different specialties
    - Dealing with varied patients (age, social background, etc.)
    - Dealing with different activities (prevention, treatment, practice management and administration, home visits)
- More flexibility to accommodate work-life balance
- Early contact and responsibilities with patients as training is quicker than for hospital doctors
- Provides many opportunities for people with an entrepreneurial drive (as GP practices nowadays operate as businesses)
- Usually attracts more friendly, caring doctors who enjoy communication and working in broad teams.

Physician (sometimes also called "Medic")
This is the term used for doctors who have a preference for the diagnostic and medical treatment of patients (as opposed to surgical treatment).

- Usually specialised. More thorough in their approach because they have in-depth knowledge and experience of one specialty
- Enjoy intellectual challenge of dealing with complex conditions
- Approach is more pathology orientated
- Approach requires more investigations and is often empirical
- Attracts doctors who are good communicators, who enjoy working in teams, are conscientious and enthusiastic.

Surgeon
- Enjoy immediate results
- Increased patient satisfaction due to more immediate and "dramatic" results of surgery
- More procedure orientated. Surgery attracts doctors who have good dexterity (obviously!) and have a keen eye for detail
- Requires patience and endurance
- Being a more competitive environment, people who do well in surgery tend to be more dynamic and decisive.

How to approach the question

Your preference will have originated from your work experience or from other settings. Therefore, you must use your own experience of Medicine to explain your point of view.

You should also ensure that you describe what made you interested in that particular section of Medicine, rather than simply state that you found it "interesting, fascinating, enlightening or enriching".

Finally, make sure that you have a sentence that presents you as broad-minded and that you have set your heart on a realistic career. If you go too strongly for one aspect of Medicine or, even worse, one of the many specialties (e.g. cardiology), they will simply counter you by saying: "How do you know you will like it for 40 years when you have observed it for only 2 weeks?!"

Example of an effective answer

During my work experience, I was fortunate to observe a cardiologist, a GP and a urologist. During that time, I observed a lot of similarities but also some differences in the approach to patient care. I must say I enjoyed my surgical attachment more than the other two. I was particularly motivated by the competence with which the surgeon treated the patients.

Also, although the ward rounds were very busy, he took time to teach both the nurses and me. I observed the way he communicated with his patients and the rest of the team. His approach was clear and decisive.

More importantly, I was very encouraged by how quickly the patients recovered after the surgery and that really inspired me to think about a career in surgery as I feel I would get personal satisfaction out of my job.

Having said that, I do recognise that I still have plenty to learn about the system and my time at medical school will give me a good opportunity to learn about and reflect on each career option so that I can make a fully informed decision once I have graduated.

Another example of an effective answer

Most of my work experience was spent in a hospital shadowing a cardiologist. It really taught me a lot about the manner in which physicians approach their patients. I was particularly impressed by the wide range of skills that the consultant and his colleagues possessed. Having a very analytical mind, I enjoyed observing their problem-solving approach when they had to diagnose a patient.

I also witnessed the crucial role that communication plays in a physician's day. Not only did they have to explain complex conditions to patients who had no medical knowledge, they also acted as counsellors and, in some cases, needed to show a lot of care, attention and empathy. As someone who enjoys working in close contact with people, I found this proximity to the patient very appealing and, in that regard, I feel that I would enjoy being a physician.

Obviously, my time at medical school will give me many opportunities to become familiar with other career options and at this stage I would like to keep an open mind.

And another...

One of my main motivations for getting into Medicine has been the work that I did in Southern India, working for 2 months in a rural community, helping women give birth in really difficult conditions. Although it was sometimes difficult to deal with, I really enjoyed the obstetrics work and this is something that I would really like to do as a career.

Back in the UK, I had the opportunity to shadow an Obs & Gynae consultant for 2 weeks and this has only reinforced my desire to get into an obstetrics career. As well as the extreme feeling of satisfaction that I got from helping a baby being delivered, I enjoyed enormously the buzz of working on busy labour wards when I was there.

Having said that, my current choice of career is only based on my experience so far and I am sure that medical school will give me lots of opportunities to experience the good sides (and maybe the not-so-good sides) of other specialties. Therefore I might be better placed to answer this question in a more definite manner in 5 years' time once I have graduated.

7.10 What do you want to achieve in your medical career?

The CAMP structure will give you a good framework for your answer.

- **Clinical;** you will want to develop a strong career where you can excel from a clinical point of view. Maybe you already have some idea of the type of specialty that you want to pursue (see previous questions). Perhaps you have an interest in charity work and would like to use your medical skills.

- **Academic:** you may have an interest in research that originates from previous experience or exposure. You may also be interested in teaching others and will want to ensure that you develop good teaching skills during your training and beyond with the aim of playing a substantial part in the training of future doctors. You may even have thought about becoming a lecturer.

- **Management:** being a doctor is more than just being a clinician. You will want to build experience in managing and leading teams, improving and developing new services.

- **Personal:** you will want to make sure that you have a healthy work-life balance. Maybe there are activities that you enjoy greatly (hobbies, voluntary/charity work) and that you would like to pursue (don't spend too long on this; it is a slight tangent as not strictly Medicine-related, but still okay to mention).

Example of an ineffective answer

I hope to become a doctor in a busy teaching hospital treating sick patients. I want to make a difference to those patients who are in need, especially the children.

Apart from the fact it only has two sentences and will hardly fill a 2-minute slot, the above answer is ineffective for many reasons:

- It starts well by giving a clear aim, but the candidate does not explain his reasons. Why does he want to work in a busy teaching hospital rather than a District General Hospital or even become a GP? Is it because he has ambitions to be a specialist in an environment that provides many academic opportunities? Or because he wants to teach at a high level? Whatever the reasons they must be explained, for this is where the real value of his answer lies.

- "I want to make a difference to those patients who are in need" is a fairly generic statement. You could do many other jobs and still fulfil that criterion. A porter would make a difference to a patient in need. Also, he declares an interest in children, but does not really explain why he has such an interest. Has he worked with children before? Has he got any other personal experience with children in general? How is he proposing to achieve this? By specialising in paediatrics? By becoming a GP? By being a doctor in some completely different specialty but doing volunteer work for a local orphanage?

The answer needs to be explained and personalised a lot more.

Example of an effective answer

There are many things that I would like to achieve during my medical career and I am really looking forward to taking on all kinds of challenges. From a clinical point of view, I would like to build strong medical background knowledge with a view to specialising either in paediatrics or oncology. I have developed an interest in these two specialties through some of my reading as well as my work experience and I feel that working in those specialties would provide me with a career in which I can make a real difference to people's lives by showing a caring and empathic approach, and adopting a way of working which is more holistic than, maybe, other specialties.

I have also always liked teaching and training others, and have had many opportunities at school to become involved in tutoring other students. This is an interest that I would like to develop further throughout my career, and I would like to think that I could play a substantial role in the training of junior doctors both during my training and once I am fully specialised.

Outside Medicine, but still related, I want to make full use of my organisational skills to make sure that I can carry on working with the Red Cross, with which I have been involved for the past 3 years.

7.11 What are the pros and cons of being a doctor?

This question tests your general understanding of the role of doctors and how realistic your view of Medicine is. Although the CAMP structure (see Section 6.4) is not entirely appropriate here since the answer clearly has to be structured around pros and cons, you can still use it to generate ideas.

Here are examples of points you could make:

Pros
- Opportunity to use your skills to treat patients and make a difference
- Dynamic subject which requires constant learning
- Rewarding to teach the next generation of doctors
- Opportunities to get involved in activities such as research where you can contribute to medical advancement
- Opportunities to use a wide range of skills at a high level (communication, team playing, management, leadership, organisational skills)
- Respected by the public.

Cons
- Can be stressful, particularly if exposed to long hours, changing shift patterns, difficult patients, or having to make difficult decisions on your own
- May become too involved emotionally with patient care
- Some aspects of Medicine can be routine (paperwork, etc.)
- Need to manage high quality care with limited resources
- Constantly under public scrutiny. Always exposed to danger of complaints
- Patients may have unreasonable expectations
- Compromise on work-life balance because of on-calls and possible unsociable hours
- Often dealing with uncertainty.

In this question, you either come up with ideas or you don't. All you need are four or five ideas for each section that you can explain and develop briefly. Also, in order to being the answer to life and to stand out (knowing that many other candidates may come up with similar points), try to give examples from your work experience.

7.12 What are you looking forward to the most and the least about becoming a doctor?

This question is very similar to Q.7.11: "What are the pros and cons of being a doctor." By asking about both what you are looking forward to the most and the least, interviewers get a chance to test that you have insight into the fact that the future is not all rosy.

What you are looking forward to the most

Try to choose points that are of a more practical nature. You can use the CAMP structure to give you some ideas. Here are a few examples:

Clinical
- The challenge of dealing with people from different backgrounds and cultures
- Constantly developing new knowledge to keep up with medical advancement
- The chance to specialise in an area of interest (useful if you have some idea of what you want to do)
- The troubleshooting nature of Medicine and the challenge of reaching a diagnosis
- The practical nature of the work and the opportunity to take actions which have a tangible result on people.

Academic
- The opportunity to get involved in teaching or research.

Management
- The opportunity to mentor and train others
- The opportunity to develop new ideas that may lead to improvements in patient care.

Personal
- The chance to make some difference to people
- The chance to work in small and large teams
- Variety in the work
- The chance to make a difference not just through science but also through softer skills such as your empathy and communication skills.

What you are looking forward to the least

This will essentially be the same points as the cons raised in Q.7.11.

Example of an effective answer

I am passionate about the opportunity to use my skills to treat patients and make a difference. I think this is the most rewarding part of being a doctor. The ability to treat an ill patient and to watch them recover from the illness is a priceless gift.

I am also keen to continue to learn new skills in Medicine since it is a dynamic subject, which requires regular updating in my knowledge. Using this knowledge, I am keen to teach the next generation of doctors. I have strong communication skills and people management skills, and I am looking forward to using those with both patients and colleagues.

I do understand that there are difficulties in being a doctor too. I am a caring person and I guess that I will need to ensure that I do not get too involved emotionally in treating patients. I have also observed that doctors do not always have enough time or resources to attend courses to update their knowledge and to teach others, and that they are sometimes being rushed around, and I guess that this can make the job harder.

Also, there has been a lot of negative publicity about doctors and doctors are constantly under public scrutiny. This is a type of pressure that I do not particularly look forward to. However, overall I feel that there are many more advantages than disadvantages in being a doctor.

Medicine is something that I feel very passionate about and I look forward to starting my training as soon as possible so that I can experience its good sides and learn to deal with its less attractive features.

Note how the positive aspects are handled in a personal manner: "I am passionate...", "I am keen". On the other hand, the negative aspects are handled in a detached manner: "I understand ...", "I have observed..." This helps reduce the impact of the negative points and ensures that they are not perceived as being a problem for the candidate. The positive conclusion also helps in leaving a positive final impression.

7.13 Why do some students who qualify as doctors give up Medicine and never practise?

Salient points (using the CAMP structure, see Section 6.4) include:

Clinical
- They find Medicine too complex or the training too lengthy.
- Too much learning to be done before you can have responsibilities.
- They can't cope with being personally responsible for a patient's life or death.
- The exams are a burden and once you qualify there are more exams and assessments. It will take years to become a consultant.
- Dealing with patients is not as glamorous as it sounded when they first started. It can be demoralising to deal with people who complain about every little thing or people who have high expectations.

Academic
- They do not enjoy research or reading about it. It was fun as a 17-year-old but reading research papers at a more complex level is no longer enjoyable.
- They do not enjoy teaching others or get frustrated having to work with juniors who are not independent.

Management
- They feel too much time is spent on paperwork or meetings.
- They feel there is pressure to get involved in non-clinical activities such as quality improvement or service development, which takes them away from basic clinical care.

Personal
- They come from an environment where they were the best and, amongst people of a similar calibre, they do not feel that they can shine.
- They do not feel particularly ambitious and they feel uncomfortable in a competitive environment.
- Teamwork is not for them; they might prefer a profession where they can be more independent.
- Medicine is stressful. As well as long hours and big responsibilities, you have to cope with sick people all the time (including children) and death.

- Their ambitions lie elsewhere (e.g. they might have been pushed into Medicine by their parents).
- They can't multitask.
- Long hours or unsociable hours can make it difficult to have a stable private life.
- No regular pattern to life means that it can be difficult to plan and have regular hobbies.
- Some doctors change job often. This can disrupt family life.
- Health problems or personal problems.
- No real financial reward. Friends who are not doctors have a better lifestyle and more money.
- Jobs are not guaranteed. What would you do if you did not succeed to gain a position that you liked?

Delivering the answer
The question is very factual and all you need to do is develop a number of the key ideas described above. Simply list them in some kind of orderly fashion (CAMP should help you) and explain what you mean for each.

Concluding your answer
It would be a good idea to conclude the answer by reminding the panel about a few good qualities. This could be something like:

As far as I am concerned, I am a tenacious person with high ambitions. I am also very determined and well organised. This, I am sure, will help me get through the difficult times that are unavoidable.

7.14 How does Medicine now compare with 100 years ago?

Knowledge and medical advancement

- 100 years ago, there was less scientific knowledge. Doctors did not fully understand the mechanics and chemistry of the human body; they mainly treated symptoms in the best way they could but did not have the tools to get a full picture of the origins of a particular condition.

- For further information on medical advancement, refer to Section 3 on the history of Medicine.

Specialisation

- 100 years ago, doctors were mostly General Practitioners. There was not enough knowledge to have specialist doctors in many fields.

- Nowadays, there are over 60 specialties, some of which are branching out further.

Attitude towards patients

- 100 years ago, Medicine was fairly paternalistic. It also adopted a "doctor knows best" approach (the doctor was the boss and patients did what they were told).

- Nowadays, Medicine attracts a much more varied population (more women, doctors from various ethnic backgrounds, etc.). The emphasis is on patient-centred care and doctors have essentially become patient health managers. Their role is to propose. Except for a few scenarios, the final decision always rests with the patient.

Free care and formalised frameworks for regulation and probity

- 100 years ago, the NHS did not exist (created 1948) and most of the care was provided on a private basis, i.e. essentially reserved for the rich. Nowadays, care is provided more or less free of charge to everyone.

- The Royal Colleges and other institutions such as the GMC evolved to take on a regulatory role and to become the guardians of high clinical standards. Since the 1990s, this has been marked by the introduction of the clinical governance framework (see Section 5.5).

Nature of the work, role of the doctor

- 100 years ago, the emphasis was on treating symptoms. Because doctors had little understanding of diseases, there was little emphasis on prevention.

- Nowadays, and particularly since the 1980s, there is much more emphasis on prevention to deal with the more common diseases (lung cancer, cardiac diseases, skin cancer, etc.). The arrival of the internet has also facilitated the dissemination of information and therefore helped raise the level of awareness of the population.

- The doctor now has a wider role. He does not only treat patients but also gets involved in regular teaching activities. He is also required to audit his own practice and may get involved in management issues (risk management, staff management, etc.).

Revolutionary changes to the nature of diseases to be treated

- A number of major discoveries have changed the nature of the beast doctors were fighting. Vaccination has enabled humans to control a large number of common diseases and antibiotics have also radically altered the management of common infections. Coupled with a strong hygiene policy and medical advancement, this has raised the life expectancy of the population considerably. This does not come without consequences (more cancers, more geriatric diseases, etc.).

- For the most part, the UK has an affluent ageing population, which has led to the evolution of diseases "of excess" such as coronary heart disease.

- New diseases have also emerged (such as HIV/AIDS) to complicate the picture further.

Multidisciplinary approach to patient care

- 100 years ago, most doctors practised in isolation. Nowadays, the emphasis is on teamwork and a multidisciplinary approach. This involves doctors working with doctors from other specialties at all grades. It also involves working with specialists from other disciplines and associated professionals such as specialist nurses, physiotherapists, occupational therapists, dieticians and social workers.

Note that the above applies principally to the UK and other developed countries. In the developing world, the picture is different. New technologies are slowly finding their way there, but infectious diseases and malnutrition remain the main preoccupation in an environment where resources are limited.

7.15 What do doctors do apart from treating patients?

This question is designed to test your understanding of the role of a doctor in its entirety and, in a sense, the effort you have put into gaining that understanding.

What should you include?
To give a thorough answer, you can use the CAMP framework described in Section 6.4.

Clinical
- As well as treating patients' illnesses, doctors are involved in prevention work (advice on lifestyle, vaccination, etc.).
- Doctors need knowledge in order to treat patients. This is gained by attending regular teaching sessions and courses. They also take relevant exams and attend relevant seminars and conferences.
- In some cases, doctors can also be involved in counselling patients and helping them deal with the consequences of their illnesses, whether by themselves or by involving other professionals.

Academic
- Doctors spend time teaching medical students and other doctors (either junior doctors or doctors from other specialties).
- Many doctors have some involvement in research, although the degree of involvement varies depending on their specialty and the post in which they work.

Management
- Doctors may take team management responsibilities, e.g. organising rotas, organising theatre lists or clinic schedules.
- Doctors are also involved in quality improvement activities. This may include developing or improving guidelines, carrying out audits to determine if best practice is being followed and improve practice if necessary, reporting critical incidents and analysing the causes of mistakes being made so that quality of care can be improved, working on improving the experience of patients (for example by finding ways of making clinics or theatres more efficient, reducing waiting times, etc.).
- Doctors may engage in service development activities, e.g. by introducing new types of clinics or procedures.

Personal
- Since this question relates to the work of doctors, this section is not so relevant here. However, if you wish you can talk about the need for doctors to relieve stress and therefore the importance of a good social life and a few hobbies.

How to deliver the answer

This question is very much a factual question and there is no need to go overboard on selling yourself here. All they will be testing is your knowledge of the role of doctors. As such it would be enough to list a few of the activities listed below, making sure you provide sufficient variety.

If you can, in order to make the answer sound less like a list, you could illustrate the answer with events that you witnessed during some of your work experience. For example:

Doctors spend time reflecting on their clinical practice. For example, when I shadowed a gastroenterology junior doctor this summer, he spent some time collecting data for an audit designed to check that his department complied with a given national guideline. That audit led to the department changing the way it sought consent for patients before a procedure.

or

When I spent time at my local GP practice, the senior partner organised a meeting once a week with the whole team where they could discuss the difficulties that each member of the practice, whether a doctor, a nurse or a receptionist, had encountered during the previous week. That enabled them to identify areas that could be improved or where particular members of the team needed more support. In turn that helped improve staff morale and the level of the service provided.

7.16 What is holistic medicine?

This term is used extensively nowadays. In an era when patients are placed at the centre of the care, doctors must find ways of addressing their needs from various angles.

Holistic medicine means that you are treating the patient as a whole, i.e. not only the physical aspect but taking into account social, psychological and spiritual issues. Examples of holistic medicine include the following:

- A patient has a rash. An easy option would be to give him an ointment to apply to rid the patient of that rash. A holistic approach would be to determine whether this rash may have a psychological origin or be due to a stressful lifestyle. On top of providing treatment for the rash, the doctor would assist the patient in overcoming those other issues. He would also study how the rash and the treatment affect the patient's life, work and self-esteem, and would ensure that any negative effects are minimised.

- A patient has been diagnosed with a chronic illness such as multiple sclerosis. As well as helping the patient to cope with the physical aspects of the illness, the doctor would consider the psychological impact of the illness on the patient and on the family. He would also consider the implications of the illness on the patient's social life, including financially, and any modifications that may need to be made to help the patient to cope effectively. A condition with long-term deterioration may have a significant impact on an individual.

7.17 How important is Information Technology (IT) in Medicine?

This question calls for a little bit of lateral thinking and some awareness of changes that are taking place in the NHS, rather than for any particular technique.

In order to produce a complete answer, you must avoid thinking about the question randomly (or panicking because IT is not your forte), and you must start thinking about the topic in an orderly and logical fashion, using the different settings in which IT may be used.

Doctors and clinical work

- Doctors use word processing to send referral letters, produce reports or prepare educational material.

- Many GP practices and hospitals store patient data on computers, making it easy to retrieve.

- Some units are linked to external systems, enabling fast transmission of information. For example, a pathology lab could post the results of a blood test onto a system, which can then be accessed remotely by doctors working in a different area, providing fast access. Also, radiologists can have X-rays and scans sent to their home or secondary place of work electronically for reporting. The need to be on-site is greatly reduced, which makes the process more efficient. Some hospitals even have their X-rays sent to Australia overnight so that a doctor can write a report, meaning that the report is available the next morning when they get to work.

- Doctors have far easier access to information, making it easier to keep up to date about recent developments. Essentially information can simply be accessed through downloads rather than having to read countless printed journals.

- Doctors can use media such as email to request advice from others, making it easier to obtain expert advice from colleagues (who can sometimes be in a different hospital and even a different country).

- Recent developments have shown new organs could be built using a 3D printer.

Doctors and other work

- Doctors can use IT to analyse data, for example as part of a research or an audit project. This produces faster and more accurate results.

- Doctors can use IT for teaching purposes, not only by using slides in presentations, but also through the use of simulators (e.g. in surgery).

Patients

- Patients can often make GP appointments and ask for repeat pre-scriptions online, making it easier to access services.

- Patients can choose where they want their care to be provided. When choice is made available, patients can often log onto a system to make that choice. This saves on paperwork.

- IT, particularly the internet, provides endless information to patients. This makes them more informed (and sometimes misinformed) and drastically affects the expectations patients have of their doctor.

7.18 As a doctor, who would you regard as part of the team?

This is a small trick question to test whether you have an open or obtuse view of the medical environment. Essentially, you must look at the concept of "team" in its broadest sense.

Immediate team

- Other doctors working with you, senior and junior
- Nurses and healthcare assistants
- Managers (bed managers, ward managers, practice managers)
- Secretaries and receptionists
- Other staff such as radiographers.

Peripheral team

These are people who you work with but may not be with you all the time:
- Doctors from other wards if working in hospital
- GPs (if working as a hospital specialist)
- Hospital specialists (if working as a GP)
- Dieticians
- Porters
- Physiotherapists
- Occupational therapists
- Social workers
- Police (in some cases)
- Community doctors and nurses
- Managers.

And of course

- Patients, who should be involved at all stages in their own care.

There is no real technique for this question, other than making sure that you mention people from all walks of life, that you do not forget patients and that, for each type of colleague, you mention what role they play in the team. Using examples from your own work experience would also be a bonus.

7.19 How important is teaching in the medical profession?

There is only one answer to this question, which is that it is vitally important since this is what enables doctors to progress through their careers by acquiring new knowledge and learning new skills.

Doctors are involved in teaching in different ways. They can:

- Supervise other doctors on a day-to-day basis and provide guidance as and when necessary.
- Help prepare junior doctors for exams through teaching classes and mock exams.
- Organise departmental teaching sessions.
- Give presentations to other doctors, both within and outside their place of work (e.g. at conferences).
- Teach in theatre through observation, demonstrations and practice. Surgical teaching can also involve the use of mannequins and videos.

Teaching is important because:

- It helps doctors and associated professionals develop new skills and build their career.
- Good teaching promotes better knowledge, better skills and therefore better patient care.
- It enables the team to spend time together away from day-to-day activities. This can help create bonds between individuals and therefore promotes team spirit.

7.20   Who should a doctor teach?

Another very factual question where you need to demonstrate a breadth of understanding of what a doctor does.

Doctors should have the responsibility of teaching the following people:

- Medical students
- Junior and senior doctors from their close team
- Doctors from other specialties and GPs
- Nurses
- Paramedics
- Healthcare workers such as dieticians, physiotherapists, social workers
- Administrative staff such as secretaries and managers
- Patients, on disease management and healthcare issues.

Do not forget the patients and, if you can, give examples of teaching situations you have come across during your work experience.

7.21 When you are a doctor, would you like to get involved in teaching?

This question is almost a trick question because whether you like it or not you will have to get involved in teaching in one way or another.

In answering the question, you should of course put across your enthusiasm for teaching, highlighting any experience of teaching that you have gained whether by helping others do their homework, or presenting in front of a group of people, or otherwise. In addition, it is important that you mention why you enjoy teaching (it is rewarding to see others progress through your own efforts; teaching facilitates teamwork and it also enables you to learn through your preparation).

Example of an effective answer

Teaching is an activity that I know I will enjoy and that I would very much like to pursue as a doctor. I have always been involved in teaching in one way or another.

As a child and a teenager, I was always involved in supervising my little sister during her homework, answering her questions and explaining to her difficult concepts in different ways. More recently, I have presented a number of topics to my class, including one on green energy and one on enzymes. I really enjoyed the preparation for the presentation as well as the delivery. I had made sure that I knew my subject well and, as a result, the feedback was that everyone found the talk and the question and answer session very informative.

What I enjoy about it is the fact that you are able to make someone's knowledge evolve through your own work and that you do learn quite a lot from it yourself.

7.22 Do you know what it's like to be a medical student?

This question is not only about your idea of what the next 5 years will be like but also about how you found out about it. This would include open days, talking to students and lecturers, reading the prospectus, visiting the school's website, etc. You need to present a balanced view of medical school but, ultimately, you must make sure that you emphasise the work required and the skills needed more than the social aspect.

Example of an effective answer

Nobody can really say that they know what it is like to be a medical student if they have not been through medical school themselves; however, having spoken to many people and read up on it, I feel that I have a good idea of what is awaiting me.

It is no secret that medical school is hard and can sometimes be stressful. All the students I have talked to during the open day have mentioned this as the biggest step that they have had to overcome. There are many lectures and workshops to attend, homework and personal studies to undertake, presentations to prepare and generally an awful lot of information to assimilate.

On top of this we all come from an environment where we have been spoon-fed a lot and we are going into an environment where we have to think for ourselves, which requires a lot of personal skills and resilience.

As a medical student, you have to know how to work in teams. You also have to know how and when to take the initiative and take leadership in the projects that you are handling. You also need to keep your knowledge up to date by reading up on issues and finding your own information. Being someone who is very organised and meticulous, I am ready for all this.

At the same time, I also have a number of personal interests, which will enable me to deal with the pressure and stress involved. I intend to continue to pursue my sporting interests in football and rowing with my new friends at university.

7.23 What are the extended roles of nurses in healthcare?

The issue of "extended roles of nurses" has become increasingly topical and is causing many controversies. We will deal with these in the next question.

Generally speaking, you must be very careful to consider nurses respectfully as there may be one on the panel and, in any case, it is always good to demonstrate a little bit of respect and team spirit towards people with whom you will be working. During your medical career, nurses will greatly contribute towards your education and your ability to care for your patients effectively.

Background

The introduction of the European Working Time Directive has led to a decrease in the number of working hours for doctors. The overall impact is that more doctors are needed to care for patients; this has encouraged the profession and the government to take a number of steps.

One of these steps has been to recognise that some of the tasks traditionally performed by doctors could actually be done by other people if these people were adequately trained. Similarly, a number of patients could be seen by other health professionals instead of doctors. As a result, some nurses have been able to take on an extended role.

How have nurses' roles been extended?

The main areas nurses are involved in are:

- *Clinical nurse practitioners in specialist fields*
  These are nurses who have a lot of experience in one specialty and can take on some of the duties traditionally performed by doctors in that specialty. This could involve running specialist clinics, following up on patients previously seen by a doctor, and even doing minor operations or procedures. These nurses can take histories and examine patients, carry out investigations, and prescribe drugs (within limits set down by protocols and signed off by consultants). Nurses can also run walk-in centres where they can make decisions about acute patient care. There are several grades, running up to "nurse consultant".

- **Nurse managers**
  These are nurses who have taken on a managerial role; for example, recently, we have seen the reintroduction of matrons on wards. In the community, there are nurses who are responsible for managing other nurses over an entire region.

- **Research nurses**
  A small number of nurses are involved in research activities.

See Q.10.32 for the advantages and disadvantages of the increasing role of nurses.

7.24 Does the bulk of medical treatment occur in the community or in hospital?

The short answer is: in the community.

Your reasoning should include:

- Many people self-medicate. You do this when you buy any drug without prescription at your local pharmacy or supermarket.

- GPs are the obligatory first port of call and many people do not go on to see a specialist following a GP consultation.

- Gradually, GPs have started to develop special interests (diabetes, dermatology, ophthalmology, minor surgery, etc.) and actually provide basic specialist care in clinics at their practice. This further reduces the burden on hospital doctors.

- A large number of patients have chronic diseases (asthma, diabetes, arthritis, etc.). Once the patient has been seen by a specialist, the care is often transferred to the GP, who will monitor and manage the treatment. Treatment may then be either self-administered or provided by community nurses.

- There are specialist doctors such as community paediatricians or community psychiatrists who provide treatment in the community.

- Hospital specialists are encouraged to run "outreach" clinics, i.e. beyond the hospital site.

  Overall, hospital treatment actually covers a small proportion of medical treatment. The government is currently pushing to substantially increase the amount of care being provided in the community and this trend can therefore only grow.

| 7.25 | **Why is research important in Medicine?** |

A very factual question that requires an answer with a bit more depth than the often quoted: "Because we can discover new things". One could probably write entire books about this topic but in 2 minutes you will need to come up with something practical and simple.

Research is, of course, important for the advancement of Medicine as it enables doctors and private institutions to derive new techniques, new technology and new drugs that all contribute to better care for patients.

Research leads to publication and the build-up of knowledge that can then be used to improve standards of care in Medicine. This process of analysing information and evidence derived from research and applying one's clinical judgement to make it relevant to individual patients' situations is called Evidence-Based Medicine.

Research can take many forms. It can be lab-based, or patient-based, or even sometimes simply literature-based (i.e. analysing the different pieces of literature existing on a particular topic and drawing conclusions from it).

Once you have briefly explained what research is about (keeping it nice and simple), you can conclude by saying that it is something that you take an interest in (give the names of a few articles that you read recently) and that you look forward to getting involved in research projects at some stage as a doctor.

7.26	If a benefactor offered you a large amount of money to set up a Medical Research Centre and invited you to run it, what area of research would you choose to invest in and why?

To answer this question well, you have to demonstrate some degree of knowledge in scientific subjects. Doing some reading on scientific advances and keeping up to date with current news will help you give a meaningful and more detailed answer.

It is generally better to talk about diseases that have high impact, such as HIV/AIDS, breast cancer or multiple sclerosis, rather than something too specialised, where you run the risk of being asked awkward questions about a topic that you know little about. If, however, you have good knowledge of a more obscure condition, for example because you know someone who has been affected by it, then you should go with it.

When you deliver the answer, bear in mind that the point of this question is not to ascertain your actual research interest (by the time you become a senior doctor, Medicine will have vastly moved on from where it is today), but to determine that you have an interest in medical issues. So, make good use of your reading material and personal interests.

Example of an effective answer

I think one of the exciting fields in Medicine at the moment is the possible use of vaccines to cure cancer. I have recently read about the randomised control trials in treating cervical cancer. I really think that this is an exciting field in Medicine. The fact that vaccines were developed to prevent the infection of HPV virus and subsequently have the potential to cure cervical cancer is a real breakthrough. This vaccination technique has the potential to lead to cures for common cancers such as prostate and breast cancer.

Of course, this may also be the answer for developing a vaccine in a devastating disease such as HIV/AIDS. This is why I would probably choose this area as a possibility for a new research project.

7.27 What has been the most important discovery in the last 100 years?

This question is tricky because it implies that there is a single answer to it. In reality, there are numerous discoveries that have made a real difference in their own way and which have all been very important (see Section 3 on the history of Medicine). Events you could mention include:

- Penicillin (in the 1940s) has revolutionised surgery by considerably lowering the risk of infection. It has been complemented by high-level advances in anaesthesia, which makes surgery what it is today.

- The invention of keyhole surgery, which has further reduced the need for invasive surgery, enabling patients to minimise the length of hospital stay and increase their chances of a quick recovery.

- Radiography in 1896. This has since been complemented by the invention of MRI scanning and other scans, which enable quick and non- or minimally-invasive diagnosis.

- Discovery of DNA by Watson and Crick in the early 1950s. Some important applications in Medicine, but also forensic science.

- The discovery of new HIV medications or combinations, which have helped transform HIV/AIDS into a chronic disease thus helping control an epidemic.

Ultimately, your choice is vast but make sure that you quote a discovery that has had a wide-ranging impact across society rather than something obscure.

In addition, you would be well advised to ignore discoveries whose application has yet to be fully understood. For example, the Genome project has undoubtedly been an important step in Medicine but its practical applications have yet to be fully appreciated. Many candidates have been caught out by a hostile reception from interviewers at the mention of the Genome project, because it has not yet yielded great returns in terms of medical advancement. The same applies to stem cell research, another favourite of medical school applicants.

7.28 What type of research would you be interested in doing?

This question can be asked to everyone. If you have already done some research in the past, then you could use the opportunity to discuss the research that you have already done and finish off by saying that you would be keen to continue exploring that field, or some other field that you identified as interesting on the way.

If, however, you have not done any research at all until now (which will be the case for many candidates), then you should concentrate on a field of Medicine that interests you, or on a topic that maybe you have read about recently.

This question is really about testing your curiosity and interest in the un-known as well as your motivation for Medicine. Therefore, your answer should set out a topic that interests you. It should explain how you become interested in that topic, and what results research could achieve in that area. The more you can use your answer to demonstrate that you are well read and well informed, the more you will impress your interviewers.

Example of an effective answer

I have always been interested in molecular biology. I really believe the potential is endless.

Molecular biology can help us, first of all, to understand the normal physi-ology. From the norm, we can then find out more about the disease proc-esses. This can, of course, point us in the direction of finding a cure for cancer, genetic conditions and AIDS.

Therefore, for the final year at medical school, I am hoping to be involved in a project in either physiology or pharmacology. I understand this univer-sity is very active in projects such as the molecular basis of multiple scle-rosis and Alzheimer's disease and I hope to be actively involved in this field in the future.

Another example of an effective answer

In the last decade of the 20th century, scientists finally cracked the genetic code as part of the so-called Human Genome Project, but it is fair to say that, since then, there has been little progress made to convert that phenomenal discovery into tangible solutions to problems. At the time, everyone talked about "the end of cancer" with great enthusiasm. Of course there has been some progress and the current trials that are taking place to see if an engineered virus can be used to heal the damaged and struggling hearts of heart failure patients are testimony to that. But that is only the start. That would be an area that would interest me greatly.

7.29 — What has been the greatest public health advance since the start of the 20th century?

Similarly to Q.7.27., the choice is vast and there is no right answer. All you need to do is demonstrate an awareness of some of the key issues. Note that the question is asking about a public health advance (i.e. something that affected the whole population) and not just a medical advance.

Here are a few examples:

- Introduction of the NHS in 1948

- Eradication of smallpox and polio

- Invention of antibiotics in the 1940s

- Better family planning – family planning altered socioeconomic role of women, reduced family size, increased birth intervals, and improved maternal and child health; barrier contraceptives also reduced unwanted pregnancies and transmission of sexually-transmitted diseases

- Fluoridation of drinking water – resulted in reductions in tooth decay and tooth loss

- Safer and healthier foods – decrease in microbial contamination and increase in nutritional content; nutritional deficiency diseases (rickets, goitre, pellagra) almost eliminated

- Decline in deaths from coronary heart disease and stroke – from risk-factor modification (especially smoking cessation and blood pressure control) and improved access to early detection and treatment

- Recognition of tobacco use as a health hazard and subsequent smoking ban in public places – resulted in changes in social norms, reduced prevalence of smoking and mortality from smoking-related diseases

7.30 What challenges do you think a career in Medicine will pose to you? How will you deal with them?

Because this question relates to your experience of Medicine, you can use the CAMP structure (see Section 6.4) to build your answer. The question refers to "challenges" and so, as you deliver the answer, you will need to ensure that you indicate why each point is a challenge and that you use the opportunity offered to you to explain how you can surmount them. Here are examples of points that you can make:

Clinical

- Training as a doctor is, in itself, a challenge. You need to study hard and pass exams. This takes endurance and hard work.

- As a junior doctor you will face situations that you cannot necessarily handle. In many cases, you will be able to ask for help; but there may be situations where you may be challenged. In such situations you will also need to manage patients' expectations and maintain their faith in you.

- As a doctor there will inevitably be situations where you make mistakes or, at least, do not act as well as you could have. You will need to be brave to confront such situations, be honest about your mistakes and ensure you learn from them. This requires integrity and a strong willingness to learn and to develop. This will require honesty and good communication skills.

- You may need to make difficult decisions at very short notice, for example when dealing with acute emergencies. Some of your decisions may be a matter of life and death. To achieve that you will need to be decisive but also always remain safe in the way you make decisions.

- As a student and as a doctor, you will constantly need to develop your knowledge. Medicine evolves constantly and it is crucial that you keep up to date. This can be challenging when so much literature is available and you spend a lot of time dealing with patients. Although keeping up to date can be done by attending one-off formal events such as courses and conferences, you will also need to read journals, and attend and run departmental teaching, all of which takes time. This will require discipline and an appetite for knowledge.

- You will be facing challenges from patients themselves. Some will be demanding; others won't care. Some will bore you with too much information; others will be too succinct or will withhold information Some will be eloquent; others won't even speak English. Some will have a culture and behaviour to which you can relate; others will be so different to you that you may struggle to understand their reactions. Dealing with such challenges will require patience, good communication skills, empathy, and an ability to be open-minded and non-judgemental.

- As part of your clinical work you will need to work with other colleagues, some more junior than you, some more senior; some from your own specialty, others from different specialties or other types of professions (e.g. porters, technicians, nurses, midwives, managers). You will need to get along with everyone despite everyone pushing their own agendas. There are times when you may face real conflict; for example, a radiologist may refuse to perform a scan that you ordered because he/she doesn't think it is appropriate; or a ward doctor may refuse to admit a patient whom you think should be admitted. Keeping focused on the patient's needs, demonstrating tact and showing good team playing abilities will be key.

Academic

- As well as dealing with patients, you may have to get involved in teaching and research activities. These can be demanding and take time.

- Research can be a frustrating process. You can spend a lot of time to find nothing of interest.

- Teaching can also be frustrating. You may have to teach people who aren't as interested in the topic as you are.

Management

- You will need to be proficient at management, as if it wasn't hard enough to deal with the clinical side of the work.

- You will need to learn to manage people and resources. Some of those people may be more experienced than you (such as senior nurses).

Personal

- You will have to work in busy environments and during unsocial hours. This can be tiring. It requires stamina and good organisation. You will need to be able to cope under pressure to deal with stress. Part of that will involve maintaining a good work-life balance.

- Training might take you round many different hospitals. Changing area often can be disruptive to family life.

- The pattern of work can be varied. It is not a 9-5 job. You might spend some weeks on nights and others on day shifts. You may have to work some weekends.

Delivering the answer

- Choose three or four points from the list above (you can add your own) and explain how each can be a challenge as a doctor. If you can, give examples of situations from your work experience.

- Talk about the skills you possess that will help you deal with those challenges. For example:

  - If you mention that Medicine requires constant learning, and an ability to combine that with a heavy clinical workload, talk also about how you demonstrated great stamina, concentration and resilience when you had to study for your A levels at the same time as having to manage a range of other issues. Talk also about how effective you are at organising your time.

  - If you mention that you will need to deal with difficult patients, explain that you are a very patient, calm, empathic and open-minded person and give an example of a situation when you demonstrated those skills.

7.31 Tell us about something that you read about recently, which is medically related

As part of your preparation for the interview, and for entry into Medicine generally, you should ensure that you have familiarised yourself with current issues within the medical field at scientific, ethical and political levels. To do so, you don't need to spend hours reading complex publications such as *Nature* or *The Lancet* (to be honest, the interviewers will question your sanity if what you have read is well beyond your level of comprehension). You can get much of the information you need from more accessible sources such as:

- The Student BMJ (http://student.bmj.com)

- The NHS choices website – Health News section (http://www.nhs.uk/News/Pages/NewsIndex.aspx)

- The BBC's health news section (http://www.bbc.co.uk/news/health/)

and generally the health section of any major newspaper and news website.

If you have developed an interest in a particular condition either because you, or someone you know, is affected by it, or because you have come across it during your work experience, you may also want to read specialist websites linked to that condition. The most accessible specialist websites tend to be run by charities, because they seek to explain all complex issues and treatments in a language that is accessible to the vast majority of patients.

If your personal statement mentions the name of a particular condition and/or if your work experience involved caring for a particular type of patient, the interviewers will expect you to have a reasonable amount of knowledge on that topic; as such you will have no choice but to read the relevant specialist websites as there is a strong probability that you will be asked about it at your interview.

Finally, rather than asking about something that is "medically related", the interviewers may specify that they want you to talk about an ethical problem or a scientific advancement, so make sure that you have an answer prepared for different variations of the question.

What topic should you choose?

- **Scientific topics**
  A scientific topic will be appropriate if you are interviewing for one of the more academic medical schools (e.g. Oxford, Cambridge, UCL or King's) or if you have a particularly good understanding of the issues, for example through personal experience.

  Only choose a scientific topic if you are well versed in it. For example, if you want to discuss the latest advances in treating a specific condition, make sure you are able to explain what causes the condition, how it affects the patient, what different treatments are available and what their pros and cons are, how the new treatment works exactly and why the new treatment will make a difference. Avoid choosing a scientific topic if your knowledge is too superficial as you will not be able to withstand further questioning. In particular, don't mention topics for effect (e.g. stem cell research is a classic at medical school interviews).

  Finally bear in mind that you may actually be more knowledgeable on the topic than your interviewers. For example, if your two interviewers are a medical student and a cardiology consultant, they may have limited knowledge of the latest advances in cancer treatment. As such they will be relying on you to explain the issues clearly, so choose a topic that is not too technical and don't assume that they will fill the blanks for you.

- **Ethical topics**
  An ethical topic is a safe bet because the issues are never very clear cut and the topic usually lends itself to easy discussions. It also has the benefit of being understandable by interview panel members of all backgrounds. There are usually plenty of those in the news, so try to pick something fairly recent.

- **Political topics**
  Political topics (e.g. "privatisation of the NHS", service and budget cuts) are also always in the news but are far more difficult to handle than ethical topics because of the controversy that surrounds them. No matter how balanced your view may be, those on the panels may have very set views on the topic that you raise and you run the risk of alienating your interview panel without actually doing anything wrong. I would suggest you steer clear of politics if you can.

7.32 What are the causes of aggression, anger or stress in a hospital environment?

This question does not require specific knowledge of the hospital environment, and you should be able to get most of the points simply by using your own experience as a patient, and common sense.

Patients can be aggressive, angry or stressed for many reasons:

- They are under the influence of alcohol or drugs.
- They have forgotten to take medication that made them more sedate.
- They are in pain.
- They feel they are waiting too long (e.g. in A&E).
- The medical team is running late and there is a substantial delay in clinic appointments.
- Nurses and doctors are not giving them what they want (e.g. a patient demands a scan, but the staff refuse it because they feel a scan is inappropriate).
- They do not understand what they are being told.
- They do not feel that they are being listened to. Their concerns are not being addressed adequately.
- The patient has not been offered the relevant options to choose from.
- The doctors are not spending enough time with them.
- The patient feels that they are not respected, e.g. the medical staff is rude, treats the patient "like a number" or appears dishonest.
- There is confusion or conflict between what different people are telling them.
- They are scared about their diagnosis and prognosis.
- They refuse to accept what they are being told (e.g. a patient may be angry at a diagnosis of HIV or cancer and takes it out on the staff).
- The medical staff has made a mistake.
- The medical staff refuses to acknowledge that they have made a mistake.

If you have personal experience of these types of problems then give appropriate examples. It is also worth mentioning in your answer that most of the complaints in the NHS are linked to poor communication, which should be easy to resolve with proper training, care and attention, without having to spend much money.

8 Questions on the course and the Medical School

8.1 Why do you wish to study at this medical school?

The mistake often made by candidates is to massage the ego of the interviewers by telling them that there is nothing better in the world than their school, that it has a superb reputation and that it is a well-known centre of excellence. Say that in Cambridge and they will ask you why not Oxford. Say that in Manchester and they will ask you why not Leeds. You can't win. In truth, medical schools often have similar features to others and all think that they are really good. So, if you want to have an answer that sounds different to the other candidates, you will need to back up your arguments with a few facts. And that means doing some homework. Ultimately, as ever, what really matters is that you have a handful of well-chosen and well-explained reasons rather than a long list of superficially addressed bullet points.

You may find the following questions useful to define your reasons:

Course structure

- Do you prefer an integrated course or a course with 2 years of preclinical and 3 years of clinical?
- Does the school offer the opportunity to intercalate a BSc?
- Does the school offer the opportunity to get involved in research activities?
- Do you prefer a system-based approach (i.e. where you learn everything relevant, for example, to the digestive system or the respiratory system) or a subject-based approach (i.e. where you learn everything about anatomy, pharmacology, pathology and biochemistry separately)?
- Does the medical school offer the opportunity of going on an elective?

Teaching style

- Does the school offer problem-based learning (PBL) or traditional teaching?
- Are there opportunities to take up special study modules (SSMs)?
- Does the school offer dissection sessions (i.e. where you can practise yourself) or prosection (i.e. where you watch an experienced anatomist do the dissection)?
- Does the school have facilities for computer-based learning?
- Does the school offer early contact with patients (e.g. either because it is an integrated course, or because you are given an opportunity to follow some patients up)?

Associated hospitals and population

- What is the reputation of the associated hospitals?
- Do the local hospitals have strengths which match some of your specific interests?
- Is the local patient population suitably varied?
- Does the medical school provide access mainly to teaching hospitals, district general hospitals or a good mix of both? (Teaching hospitals don't always deal with huge numbers of common cases.)

Location/Social

- Do you prefer a campus or more independence?
- Is the medical school in a city centre or not?
- Is the medical school over just one site or several sites (several sites may offer more variety but may cause transport issues and time wasting)?
- Does the medical school offer student accommodation? Will you be with people from outside Medicine at the residence hall?
- Do you have friends or family in the area?
- Does the area offer facilities which suit you (e.g. access to international airport if you often need to travel abroad, easy access to areas of natural beauty, proximity to London but still in the countryside, proximity to the sea, etc.)?
- Does the school offer social activities that you enjoy such as sports or music clubs, rowing, choir, trekking and rambling, drama?

Example of an effective answer

There are several reasons why I want to study here.

I have done a lot of reading and attended the open day a couple of months ago; and one of the things that really attracted me to the school is the fact that it uses a dual approach to teaching, with a nice mix of PBL and lecture-based teaching, which means that we can approach most topics from both a theoretical and a practical perspective. I also like the fact that the school runs regular workshops, which will really provide good support to ensure that we assimilate the information. This was one of the features that the students I met at the open day preferred. Obviously, it matters a lot to me that the school is located near XXX hospital, which is a large tertiary centre of great renown as it will create good opportunities for me to see many different types of conditions and patients.

On top of that, I have also done a lot of research into the pros and cons of dissection versus prosection, which led me to conclude that prosection would most likely be a more focused way of learning anatomy; so the fact that this school offers prosection is a real bonus for me.

From a social point of view, one of my great passions in life is singing. I am currently a member of a good classical choir in my home town and I was attracted by the range of musical options that the school offers in its list of clubs.

Finally, having spent a few days in the area since I applied, I have had the opportunity to visit both the town of XXX and its region. I really enjoyed the nice mix of small historical market towns, big city centres and the easy access to the sea.

All in all, I think that the YYY medical school provides an excellent setting to study Medicine for 5 years and I am sure that I will enjoy it greatly.

8.2 There are other universities with the same teaching methods. Why this one in particular?

If you are pushed in this way, it is because they are trying to test your motivation. If you say "You are right, I don't know", this would mean that your arguments are weak and that you lack confidence in your choice. The best thing to do when you are being placed on the defensive or pushed into an uncomfortable territory is to retain your cool and look at the situation rationally. The gist of your answer will be that "of course there are other schools, and of course no real university is unique; but in the end you have to apply somewhere and you tick all my boxes".

Example of an effective answer

It is true that there are other schools that may match my criteria, and in fact I have applied to some of them. Ultimately, what I am looking for is:

1. A school that has a good training programme with a good mix of teaching styles and that supports its students. From the feedback that I got, from the syllabus and from my discussions with current students at the open day, YYY medical school offers this.

2. A school where I will be involved with patients early on and you offer this.

3. A school where I will be able to get involved in activities that I enjoy and through which I will be able to meet good friends. YYY medical school has a good range on offer and is also in a setting that I will enjoy, being close to the sea and with good proximity to interesting towns and landscapes.

Out of all the schools that I applied to I feel that YYY medical school is probably the best match to all these and I feel very confident that I will enjoy my time here and that I will reward the school with good success in my studies and in my professional life once I qualify.

8.3 What attracts you the most and the least about our medical school?

The first part of the question ("the most") should be easy to answer if you have worked out an answer to Q.8.1 ("Why do you wish to study at this Medical School?").

The second part ("the least") is a bit trickier because it is negative. Once you have mentioned a number of positive aspects about the school in accordance with Q.8.1, there are several ways in which you can address the negative points.

Strategy no.1: Sitting on the fence

This is an easy but not necessarily a bad way out. You could provide an answer such as:

Obviously every school has some less attractive aspects and I will probably come across them along the course of my studies; but, judging from all the literature that I have read and the feedback that I have obtained from students here, I think it will be a very productive and exciting experience and I am looking forward to joining the school next year.

Note that, although the answer is sitting on the fence, there is an effort to justify the answer (rather than simply saying "I can't think of anything negative", which could indicate that you simply couldn't be bothered to think about anything in particular). With this answer, you are signalling to the interviewers that you have done your homework (and you give some detail of that homework). You are also showing realism in pointing out that everything has negative aspects. Finally, you are demonstrating your enthusiasm with the final part of the answer.

This answer's only disadvantage is that it is not terribly original and will not help you stand out a great deal. However, you might not want to stand out too much on this one anyway and, if you deliver it with great enthusiasm, you could have a fairly strong impact regardless. Hopefully, the good answer that you will have provided for the features that you enjoy the most will be sufficient to allow you to sit on the fence for the features that you enjoy the least.

Strategy 2: Identifying something mildly negative that will not cause a real problem

Easy targets include the teaching methods used in the school, which have positive aspects (which you find attractive) as well as negative aspects (which you have to put up with if you want to benefit from the positive aspects). For example:

- If the medical school you apply for has a PBL training structure, the obvious drawback is the lack of background knowledge such as anatomy, physiology and biochemistry prior to patient contact.

- If the medical school of your choice is traditional, i.e. it has pre-clinical and clinical curriculum, then the obvious thing to point out is the lack of patient contact in the first 2 or 3 years.

- The medical school may not be in an area that you find the most attractive, but this is more than made up by the quality of the training that you will receive.

Whatever negative aspect you want to mention, you must make sure you tell the interviewers that it also has many advantages and that therefore nothing will cause you a real problem.

8.4 What do you know about problem-based learning (PBL)? How does it compare to other forms of learning?

Problem-based learning

PBL is a teaching method used in many medical schools in the UK. It is a method whereby you "learn to learn", which, for some candidates, is a big departure from the spoon-feeding that they have been receiving until now. As the name indicates, it is problem-based, i.e. you are given a problem, scenario, issue or question to resolve. That problem is multidimensional and therefore contains a range of learning points.

The process works as follows:

1. Students are presented with a clinical scenario or problem
2. Students determine learning outcomes and objectives
3. Students decide knowledge needed to solve problem
4. Students attempt to achieve self-determined learning outcomes (individually or in small groups)
5. Tasks are allocated among group members
6. Students present their work or contribution to group
7. Further learning points might be generated
8. Information and competencies are synthesised

How it compares to other forms of learning

PBL is the opposite of lecture-based learning. Research shows that students who have been taught mainly through lectures have greater knowledge span; however, 18 months later, PBL students have retained more knowledge from their degree. PBL has also been shown to enhance inter-professional team interaction and communication skills, which is not the case with lecture-based learning.

8.5 What are the advantages and disadvantages of PBL?

This is a factual question and, as such, there is no need to apply any specific technique to answer it. You will simply be expected to demonstrate a good awareness of the pros and cons of PBL. Here are the main ones:

Advantages of PBL

- Provides a practical view of Medicine, as applied to concrete problems.
- Suits those who have initiative. Promotes entrepreneurial spirit.
- Small group teaching. More involvement from each student (whereas traditional teaching may be more passive in nature).
- Relies on teamwork. You can therefore learn from others.
- Since you will have spent time researching a topic, you will be more familiar with the details than if they had been spoon-fed.
- Can be more rewarding once you achieve your desired objective.
- Promotes team spirit.
- Facilitator makes sure that you do not go off track.
- Early exposure to real-life issues and patient contact.

Disadvantages of PBL

- Quality of the learning depends on the quality of the problems or scenarios. A badly set up PBL programme can yield little results.
- Some topics may be best taught formally.
- PBL teaching only works if, at the end of the year, you have acquired the full knowledge that you were meant to acquire. If there are gaps, you may need to complement it by attending more traditional lectures or by doing more of your own reading.
- Relies on the quality of the facilitator's input. Rigorous training is essential.
- Students who have a more academic way of learning may not feel entirely at ease.
- Your learning experience depends on the work others in the team are willing to put in. The team may be disrupted by a lazy or non-motivated student. It could also be made dysfunctional by a student who wants to go too quickly and is more interested in getting a result than in learning.

8.6 What are the advantages and disadvantages of lecture-based teaching?

This is a factual question and, as such, there is no need to apply any specific technique to answer it. You will simply be expected to demonstrate a good awareness of the pros and cons of lecture-based teaching. Here are the main ones:

Advantages of lecture-based teaching

- Suits candidates who are autonomous in their learning.
- Presents full information in a systematic basis about all systems and relevant syllabus items.
- Easy to set up.
- Ensures all candidates receive the same information.
- Provides good background before students are "released" on patients. They might benefit more from that patient contact when it takes place.
- Students drive their own learning experience.

Disadvantages of lecture-based teaching

- Provides theoretical background with no real-life application for the first few years.
- Patient contact is delayed, which may demotivate some students (who had a more practical idea of Medicine).
- Does not suit people who learn in a less structured manner.
- Sitting in on endless lectures can be boring.
- Students may be intimidated in a large theatre and may not have the courage to participate and ask questions.
- The pace of learning is regulated by a big group and, if you are not above the average, you may be at a disadvantage. Conversely, if you are towards the top, you might find it frustrating to have to comply with the average speed.

8.7 What are the advantages and disadvantages of an integrated course?

This is another factual question requiring candidates to demonstrate a basic understanding of the course structure.

An integrated course is a course where basic medical sciences are taught concurrently with clinical studies and not in separate years. Here are the main pros and cons:

Advantages of an integrated course

- Students learn in context. Irrelevant information is less likely to be included in the curriculum. The scientific knowledge is delivered at the appropriate stage.
- Students are encouraged to take a more holistic view of a patient's problems.
- Puts greater emphasis on higher learning objectives, such as application of knowledge and problem solving skills, and promotion of staff communication and collaboration.
- Students are exposed to "real medicine" at an early stage. Early contact with patients make the subjects look less dry as you can see a direct application of what you learn.
- It encourages the application of evidence-based learning.

Disadvantages of an integrated course

- A non-integrated course may provide a stronger underpinning of the scientific theories of Medicine. With an integrated course, you may be facing patients at a time when you may not know enough to feel comfortable.
- The fundamentals of a discipline might be neglected; some topics may be omitted.
- Teachers might be less enthusiastic and less comfortable when not teaching in their own discipline.

8.8   What do you know about our course? Why does it suit you?

This question is a bit narrower than "Why do you wish to study at this Medical School?" (see Q.8.1), because it focuses on the course and not the whole school. You will need to demonstrate a good understanding of the structure of the course at that particular medical school.

A good answer should discuss three or four different aspects of the course in question, presented in three or four distinct sections. For example:

- Section 1: Integrated or non-integrated
- Section 2: PBL or traditional teaching
- Section 3: Prosection or dissection
- Section 4: Features of interest such as the possibility to do an intercalated BSc.

Example of an effective answer

One of the key attractions of the course is that it is integrated and therefore it offers early patient contact. I think that the combination of formal learning and clinical work provides an ideal platform for learning because you can see the applicability of what you learn. This will appeal to both my intellectual side, and my practical side.

In the same vein, I am excited about the combination of PBL and lectures, again because it offers this mix of theory and practical, but also because it calls for a lot of team work, meaning that you don't work in isolation. I have always been a gregarious person and learn as much from concentrating on my own as I do by sharing ideas with others.

From a practical perspective, I like the fact that the course offers dissection as opposed to prosection. Though it may seem a little more cumbersome, I enjoy learning through practice and having a hands-on approach will suit me well.

Finally, the course offers opportunities to get involved in research projects and to intercalate a BSc. That will appeal to my more academic side.

9 Questions on interpersonal skills & personal insight

9.1 How would you rate your communication skills?

Rating yourself – how to start the answer

There are several answers that are commonly given but could actually count against you. Here are a few:

- *"I would give myself 8 out of 10"* – the question I would have is "What does 8 mean? Why not 9 or 10? A number by itself is meaningless. Since you will have to provide an explanation to back it up anyway, you might as well find a more effective manner to describe your level of communication skills.

- *"I would say that my skills are average (or okay)"* – if your skills are just average or okay, there are plenty of other candidates whose skills will be better than yours and who will get the place instead. Even if this is true, you simply <u>must</u> present a more positive image.

- *"My communication skills are excellent"* – other than the fact that it sounds a little arrogant, it simply cannot really be true. Even if it were true, you would want to appear a little more humble (you are applying to become a doctor after all).

Ultimately, you will need to give the feeling that your communication skills are good. You can achieve this in many ways:

- Make a simple statement pitched at the right level: *"I think that my communication skills are good"*

or

- Talk about the skills that you have developed rather than how good you are: *"Over the past few years, I have developed some good communication skills"*

or

- Talk about what other people think of you rather than what you think of yourself: *"I have always had good feedback from my colleagues and teachers about my communication skills, and during my work experience I was often complimented by the patients at the hospice about my listening abilities."*

Developing and finishing your answer

Once you have made your opening statement, you need to explain what you mean by it, i.e. what communication skills you have, how you developed them, what they help or helped you achieve, etc. Provide concrete examples to make the answer interesting. To give a complete answer that shows an in-depth understanding of communication within the medical context, you need to convey that communication is a constantly evolving skill and that, as a doctor, you will constantly improve your communication skills through your experience and formal training.

Example of an effective answer

I have always had good feedback on my communication skills both at school from my teachers and also in all the summer jobs that I have done. One of my main strengths is my listening ability, which enables me to get on well with people in all kinds of circumstances. For example, I spent quite a long time with elderly people at my local nursing home and I felt that I made a real difference to their quality of life simply by lending an empathic ear to their problems and reacting in a caring and patient manner. I have also developed a good ability to discuss ideas with people at all levels. In one of my summer jobs I was in charge of dealing with customer complaints and, although it was challenging, I found that I could avoid conflicts simply by communicating at the right level with them and explaining complex financial issues in a way they could understand. I was also at ease teaching young children in a deprived area last year, where I needed to remain patient and explain facts several times in different ways. Being a doctor requires a wide array of communication skills. I feel that I have acquired some good foundations in that respect, which I am looking forward to developing further throughout medical school and later on through my medical career.

9.2   How have you developed your communication skills?

This question is not simply about your communication skills but how you developed them. One important aspect of being a doctor is the need to keep up to date and constantly improve. This question tests your ability to do so. Like any skill, you develop communication skills through exposure to various people and situations involving these people, either by direct involvement or by observation. This includes:

- Parents
- Friends
- Teachers at school

- Doctors from work experience
- Clients during summer jobs
- Making and learning from own mistakes

Example of an effective answer

One way in which I have developed my communication skills is simply by trying different approaches and analysing what worked and what didn't. So for example, I am the last of three children and frequently found myself having to make myself heard over two siblings who were all too keen to impose themselves in a very authoritative manner. I quickly learnt that I wasn't going to win by shouting back at them and so I developed some soft methods to influence situations to my own advantage.

Recently I have greatly improved my listening skills. Over the past 2 years, I have visited elderly people in hospices where I quickly realised that they often only wanted someone to talk to as opposed to someone who would talk at them. That taught me a lot about the value of silence and of simply being there for someone without feeling the need to fill the blanks.

I also have a good ability to explain complex issues to others. Part of it comes naturally in that I have always had a good ability to summarise information; but I have also always been very attentive to the feedback that I received from my peers, my teachers and my parents.

These are just a few examples and in reality I learn about communication skills throughout my daily life by observing others and by interacting with them constantly. Communication is a difficult skill to master but I feel that I have great strengths in this area, which I am sure will contribute greatly to making me an effective doctor.

9.3 Are you an empathic person?

Can you say "no" to this?

Empathy is the ability to put yourself in other people's shoes (virtually, not physically of course). It is a crucial skill that is required of all doctors. The answer therefore has to be "yes". Again if it were as simple as this, then there would be little point in asking the question for the sake of ticking the right box. What makes you say that you are empathic? Can you give some examples?

Example of an effective answer

Empathy is a crucial part of communication and I feel that it is a personal attribute that I possess and that I have also learnt to develop over the course of my life and of my education. Empathy is something that I have demonstrated on many different occasions. I have spent time listening to friends who were discussing their personal problems with me. As well as being an attentive listener, I always try to be non-judgemental and to view the situation from their own perspective.

Also, recently, I did some work experience in a hospice. I came across a mother of two young children who was dying of cervical cancer and I will never forget the opportunity that I had to talk to her. I spent a lot of time at her bedside and with her relatives, listening to her concerns. I sensed, through what she was saying and through her body language, that she was scared of dying, scared of leaving her children and her husband behind and that she was also feeling very lonely. I put myself in her shoes and really felt how difficult this must be to deal with. Through this, I began to understand her loneliness, her anxiety and her fears. One week after she passed away, I received a letter from her relatives thanking me for my time and understanding. This really gave me a strong sense of achievement and of having made a difference.

9.4 Can you think of a situation where your communication skills made a difference to the outcome of a situation?

This question is asking for a specific example of a situation and you should therefore use the techniques described in the first section of this book, including the STARR framework (see Section 6.3). Your first task is to identify a situation where your communication skills may make a difference. This could be, for example:

- When you were part of a team organising an event and had to negotiate with your team or third parties.

- When you had to deal with a group of people that you needed to bring round to your point of view.

- A teaching experience that was particularly challenging.

- An experience with a patient during your work experience, with whom you had to show empathy, demonstrate listening skills and discuss their problems in an appropriate manner.

This list is non-exhaustive and everyone will have had some experience at some stage, even if it is not necessarily at a high level. What matters is not so much that the example is totally fascinating but that you are able to extract the full potential out of the situation by explaining how you behaved and the impact that your behaviour had on others.

Example of an effective answer

The example used in Q.9.3 can be used as it is to answer this question.

Situation/Task
Recently, I did some work experience in a hospice. I came across a mother of two young children who was dying of cervical cancer and I will never forget the opportunity that I had to talk to her.

Action
I spent a lot of time at her bedside and with her relatives, listening to her concerns. I sensed, through what she was saying and through her body language, that she was scared of dying, scared of leaving her children and husband behind and also feeling very lonely. I put myself in her shoes and

really felt how difficult this must be to deal with. Through this, I began to understand her loneliness, her anxiety and fear.

Result & personal reflection
One week after she passed away, I received a nice letter from her relatives thanking me for my time and understanding. This really gave me a strong sense of achievement and of having made a difference.

Another example of an effective answer

Situation/Task
During a project at school, we worked in groups of 5 students and had to prepare a 10-minute presentation on a controversial topic. Although we unanimously decided that a good topic would be "The measles epidemic in Wales – should parents be allowed to choose whether to vaccinate their child or not?", this led to a huge debate within the team and numerous arguments.

Action
Throughout the discussions I could see that there were two main problems that impaired progress. First of all, instead of working on presenting the various arguments, some members of the team were trying to convince the others that their view was the only correct one. I addressed that by gently reminding everyone that the point of the exercise was not to find an answer to the dilemma, but to present the dilemma to others; and by pointing out that it was, in a way, good that we all had different views because that made it easier to find content for the presentation. Secondly, some of the team members were showing total disrespect towards others, which then started to cause voices to be raised and the quieter members of the group to become marginalised. I addressed that by facilitating the discussion in a slightly more directive way (rather than a free for all) and ensuring that those who were kept at bay were given a chance to speak.

Result & personal reflection
In that situation I was able to make a difference not only by remaining calm in the way I addressed the situation, but also by acting tactfully to control the more volatile members of the team and becoming more assertive when needed. In particular I showed a good ability to get on with people with very different types of personality.

9.5 What makes you a good team player?

As you will be studying with other people and working in teams both within and outside the hospital during your career, team playing is an essential quality of a doctor and is often tested at interviews. This question is not just about showing that you understand what team playing means; it is also about demonstrating that you possess those attributes, which you can do by giving appropriate examples.

Attributes of a good team player

In essence, a good team player is someone who:

- **Understands his role in the team and how it fits within the whole picture**
  In order to get on within a team, team players must have a thorough understanding of what they need to achieve and what is expected of them. They must also understand what is expected of others so that they can work with them effectively. In Medicine, all team members must be well coordinated in order to ensure the best care for patients and it is therefore essential that everyone in the team knows what they have to do and who else is involved.

- **Treats others with respect and is supportive**
  Team players treat fellow team members with courtesy and consideration. They show understanding and provide the appropriate support to other team members to help get the job done. Effective team players deal with other people in a professional manner. Medicine is not something that you do by yourself. There will be times when you will have problems to resolve and when you will require assistance from other colleagues at all levels and it is important that you show willingness to involve others at the right time.

- **Is willing to help**
  Good team players go beyond any differences that they may have with other team members and find ways to work together to get work done. They respond to requests for assistance and take the initiative to offer help. As a doctor, you will get requests for help from all directions (juniors, seniors and even people who are external to your place of work).

- **Is flexible and adaptable**
  Good team players adapt to ever-changing situations without complaining or resisting. Flexible team members can consider different points of views and compromise when needed. They do not hold rigidly to a point of view especially when the team needs to move forward to make a decision or get something done. They must strike a compromise between holding on to their own beliefs and convictions while respecting and taking on board other colleagues' opinions. Medicine is a teamwork environment. You may have your own views about how to proceed in a particular situation and you should be prepared to defend them. However, other people may disagree and you should be prepared to at least consider their arguments. Also, you will need to constantly question your own practice (e.g. through the audit process) and you should therefore be prepared to change your ways accordingly if necessary.

- **Communicates constructively and listens actively**
  Teams need people who speak up and express their thoughts and ideas clearly, directly, honestly, and with respect for others and for the work of the team. Good listeners are essential for teams to function effectively. Teams need team players who can absorb, understand, and consider ideas and points of view from other people without debating and arguing every point. Such a team member can also receive criticism without reacting defensively. Finally, a good team member shares information with colleagues and keeps them up to date about progress on his or her assignments. Communication is key to good medical practice. With several doctors and nurses working on the same patients, there is a great need for a coordinated approach, which is only made possible through good communication.

- **Is reliable and takes responsibility and ownership of his role**
  A good team member should do everything possible to deliver his assignments on time and with the level of quality expected of him by the rest of the team. He should get things done and do his fair share to work hard and meet commitments. Others can count on him to deliver a good performance all of the time, not just some of the time. He should also be relied upon to admit his mistakes and proactively sort them out.

How to approach the question

The easiest way to handle this question is to mention the attributes that you want to convey in a clear list and give examples for each as and when you mention them. This will give an answer that combines generic and personal.

Example of an effective answer

I have been part of many teams in the past few years and one of the qualities that my team mates often comment on is that I am approachable and supportive. For example, at school, one of my friends had trouble keeping up with the content of some of the lessons, and I spent a few evenings of my own time sitting with him to take him through some of the lessons so that he could catch up with everyone else. When I shadowed an intensive care consultant last summer, there happened to be a young student nurse in the unit who was also doing some shadowing at the same time. She was finding it hard to cope with some of the cases that we were seeing there and I had a few chats with her to make sure she was okay; she later told me she would have found it hard to cope with the attachment if I hadn't shown patience and understanding towards her situation.

In a work environment, I work very hard and pull my weight. So, for example, if I am working on a project with other people and I have been entrusted with a particular task, people know that I will always deliver a good quality product on time. I am also able to show great flexibility; for example, over the summer I worked at a well-known retail outlet on Saturdays. The manager there often called me up to see if I could step in and take on more shifts to replace some of the regular staff who had gone on sickness leave and I always showed great willingness to help by taking on those extra shifts.

I am also respectful of other people and constructive in difficult situations. For example, at school I was teamed up with someone who could be qualified as lazy. I didn't just jump in to blame him for the delays we were incurring; instead I tried to adopt a constructive approach, which ensured that he delivered on time at least part of what he was supposed to do.

Overall I am able to work with a wide range of people with different personalities, and I am sure that, as a doctor, I will make full use of those skills.

9.6 Give an example where you played an effective role as a team member

As with all questions asking you to describe an example of a situation, you should use the STARR framework (see Section 6.3) to narrate a specific situation in which you were involved, highlighting the role that <u>you</u> played.

For the purpose of this question, you should make sure that you highlight skills that are relevant to team playing as described in previous questions. You do not have to discuss all aspects of team playing but developing one or two of them well would be good.

Example of an effective answer

Situation/Task
I was recently allocated the role of marketing and selling the tickets for a school concert performance. Since there were other fund-raising events happening at the same time, this proved a difficult task and I felt that it was crucial to involve the team in making important decisions in order to avoid a disaster on the day.

Action
I contacted the project manager and asked him to set up a meeting with the rest of the team. I chaired the meeting and explained in detail to my colleagues the work that I had done, the nature of the problems that I had encountered and the initiatives that I had taken to resolve them. I encouraged my colleagues to share any ideas that they had and ensured that everyone could contribute. As a group, we came up with creative ideas of selling the tickets in the local town hall and I organised for this to take place.

Result/Reflect
As a result, we managed to have a successful concert with a full audience and raised a lot of money for charity. By being upfront with the team and encouraging a good exchange of views, I ensured that we could maximise our revenue for the event.

9.7 What are the attributes of a good team leader?

Leadership is about setting objectives and ensuring that the team is on board to achieve those objectives, which itself involves many different skills. There are many definitions of leadership. One popular definition is that a leader is someone who tells people what to do but not how to do it. In other words, a leader sets a sense of direction and purpose for the team and then ensures that the team finds its own way of working and achieves the objective with the appropriate level of supervision and support. Whatever definition you wish to adopt, a good leader must be able to demonstrate that he:

- **Has clear objectives and communicates them effectively to the team**
  In order to lead a team, a leader must have a clear sense of direction, and clear objectives. A good leader is able to communicate those objectives clearly to the rest of the team so that they can take responsibility to achieve their own goals.

- **Leads by example**
  A good leader is effective only if he is being followed by his team. He must engender respect from his colleagues by showing a good example. A leader needs to be enthusiastic, competent and confident. He needs to demonstrate that he works at least as hard as he expects others to do.

- **Understands and motivates his team**
  A good leader must understand the strengths, weakness and aspirations of each team member. This enables him to share responsibilities accordingly. He motivates his team towards achievement by:

  - Praising and encouraging others
  - Rewarding colleagues (this could be through financial incentives, promotion, or by involving team members in specific projects)
  - Empowering people and giving them responsibilities and freedom
  - Making himself available.

- **Communicates and interacts well with his team**
  A good leader should listen to the input and ideas of the team and take them on board. Communicating constantly with the team is also

important for the leader to have a good idea of how the team functions, of grievances, etc., which makes it easier to anticipate and to resolve conflict.

- **Recognises the need for change and implements it and is a decision maker**
  A good leader is not static and constantly seeks new ways of working and improving. A good leader is able to take on board all the input he receives and to make a decision on that basis. He does not seek short-term popularity at the expense of achievement.

- **Is flexible**
  A good leader will adapt his leadership style to the demands of particular situations and the individuals involved. Some situations or individuals will require him to take a hands-on approach while others may require him to take a step back and be more hands off.

How to approach the question

In order to provide an effective answer, you need to describe the main qualities of a leader as explained above. You also need to bring a personal element to the answer by giving a few brief examples of situations where you have exercised leadership.

9.8 Tell me about your leadership skills

This question is asking about your skills and not about a specific situation. Therefore the best way to address it is to identify a few situations where you have been a leader, to describe those situations and identify for each how you acted as a leader. To do this, you can base yourself on the leadership qualities described in Q.9.7.

You might have noticed that there were some similarities between the attributes of a good team player and those of a team leader. Being flexible and willing to help others belongs to both, and so does communication. Do not forget to mention the attributes that are common to both as it will soften the answer a lot. If you keep talking about making decisions, setting objectives and making others work to achieve those objectives, you run the risk of appearing a little authoritarian. Balance is what you need to show.

Example of an effective answer

I have learnt a great deal about leadership in my sixth form college, where I have been given numerous opportunities to lead in sports and Duke of Edinburgh expeditions, and to play an important part in various committees. One of my strengths is the fact that I have a clear idea of what I am trying to achieve and am able to bring people on board through my own enthusiasm and by involving them at an appropriate level. I find that it is important to involve people in making important decisions so that they can give more of themselves to achieve the team goals. For example, I had to lead a cricket team through inter-school competitions and, rather than trying to impose what I felt was right, I spent time discussing various techniques with my team so that they would all buy into the final decision.

I am also an approachable person and am open to suggestions and criticism. Not only does this make people comfortable in approaching me with their own ideas but it also enables me to identify any potential issues at an early stage. One good example is when I was part of a Duke of Edinburgh expedition during which we got lost. By remaining open to suggestions, I quickly identified that a number of team members had found a suitable alternative, which the team agreed upon and which eventually got us out of the trouble we were in.

There have also been occasions where I have needed to make important decisions by myself, either because there was no consensus amongst the team after much discussion or because there was little time to act. For example, when I was a member of the social committee of my school, I had to allocate a small budget between different activities. Obviously, everyone in the team wanted as much money for their activity as possible and I needed to be fair while remaining firm at the same time. This forced me to make decisions that were sometimes unpopular but with suitable communication I was able to avoid any real conflict and to manage my colleagues' expectations.

I really enjoy working with people. Being approachable, determined and a good communicator has really helped me succeed as a leader in many situations in the past and will be a great asset for me throughout my medical career.

9.9 Are you a leader or a follower?

This question is easier than it looks. At first glance, the word "follower" appears fairly negative and suggests that you would just follow orders and not take any initiative. But if you think about it carefully, there are many occasions where you are just a follower, with someone else taking the lead. Being a follower does not mean that you are totally passive. It simply means that, although you may be playing an important role in the team, you are not the one leading it. In that respect, more or less everyone has a boss and therefore follows someone else's lead. Being a follower certainly does not preclude you from being a good team player. Therefore, rather than take offence and give a defensive answer of the type "I am a leader of course" to please the interviewers, think about the different occasions where you have been a leader and where you have not. Within that experience lies the answer to this question.

Example of an effective answer

I am a hard-working, dynamic and enthusiastic person and I always put in the maximum effort to help my team achieve the highest performance. This is something that I have achieved as a team leader but also as someone who is ready to follow someone else's lead while retaining an important role as a team member. I have learnt a great deal about leadership in my sixth form college, where I was given numerous opportunities to lead in sports and to play an important part in various committees. One of my strengths is the fact that I have a clear idea of what I am trying to achieve and am able to bring people on board through my own enthusiasm about the project and also by involving them at an appropriate level. I find that it is important to involve people in making important decisions so that they can give more of themselves to achieve the team goals. For example, I had to lead a cricket team through inter-school competitions and I spent a lot of time discussing various techniques with my team so that they would all buy into it, rather than trying to impose what I felt was right. As a team member following someone else's lead, I have always been an active and enthusiastic colleague, and all my "leaders" have always regarded me as a valuable asset in their team. I have learnt a lot from observing other people's lead and, in that respect, it is essential to know how to be both a leader and a follower.

9.10   What makes a good team?

A team needs good team members and a good team leader who can ensure the cohesion of that team. The answer to that question is therefore a summary of the previous questions on team playing and leadership. One word of warning though: you could write books about team playing and leadership. At an interview you only have a couple of minutes to make your case, so try to be selective about the aspects of team playing and leadership that you want to present, bringing in appropriate examples to make the answer interesting. Do not worry too much about the detail.

Example of an effective answer

A good team should have both a good team leader and good team members. Essentially, you need a team of people who are enthusiastic and motivated in the work that they do, and who can take responsibility to manage their own work and achieve the results that are required from them. They should also be people who are able to show some initiative. Team members also need to be flexible in their approach so that they can adapt to change and a range of circumstances. They need to communicate well with one another to exchange information, to identify problems and to ensure continuity in the work that they do. On top of that, a good team will require a good leader who can make sure that the team members remain motivated, and who encourages the sharing of ideas and discussions to resolve problems and anticipate potential areas of conflict. A good team leader will also be able to make some of the more difficult or controversial decisions and will keep the team focused on the task.

Recently, I was involved in setting up the sixth form farewell ball. I was elected President of the ball committee, which proved very successful thanks to everyone's efforts. Everyone had contributed to setting out the goal that we had in mind and therefore supported it. Everyone was also very enthusiastic and extremely hard-working. Each had a specific role in the project but everyone was able to help others out when needed. We had regular meetings to troubleshoot any arising issues and everyone really put in a lot of effort. As the leader, I delegated the work in a fair manner and I was able to make quick decisions when needed. We had the most amazing ball and the whole college was proud of our achievement.

9.11 What are the advantages and disadvantages of working in a team?

Advantages

1. Able to spread the workload through delegation to others
2. Easier to gather ideas to deal with issues as everyone can contribute
3. Can learn from others
4. Able to rely on the support of others if you require assistance
5. Achieve more by using everyone's strengths appropriately than if you do everything by yourself
6. More social environment.

Disadvantages

1. Too much input can be confusing; it can lead to conflicts and hinder the decision-making process
2. May be more difficult for some individuals to shine if the work and rewards are shared with others
3. Breeding ground for office politics
4. Not everyone is a team player. Some elements may be disruptive
5. Will only function well if there is a strong leader
6. Can be distracting to have too many people around and could affect collective performance (too many coffee breaks and gossip!).

Delivering the answer

If you simply list the advantages and disadvantages, you will give an answer that risks resembling that of others. For your answer to stand out, you need to give examples of situations where you were in teams when things went well and when they didn't.

Concluding your answer

Overall, you do not want to give a bitter feeling about teamwork and you should try to remain objective. Here is a possible example of a neutral ending: "Overall, there are as many disadvantages as there are advantages. However, a good team is really what the individuals within it make it, which is where the role of the leader becomes important in making sure that everyone is aware of and fulfils their personal responsibilities."

9.12 How do you manage your time?

Working as a doctor will require you to multitask. Not only will you have to deal with your clinical work but you will also need to find time to study and keep up to date, to teach others, to carry out other activities such as research and audits, to attend meetings, to have your own life and to deal with emergencies when required. All this requires good organisational and time management skills, hence the question.

Bringing your experience into play, you should be able to demonstrate that you:

- Plan your work properly
- Prioritise your work in order of urgency
- Maintain appropriate communication to ensure that you know what is happening and that you can allow for any changes
- Anticipate potential problems
- Allow for the unexpected if you need to
- Allow for some time to rest.

You can also talk about tools that you use to help you with your time management. This would include:

- A diary (paper or electronic)
- Making task lists (paper, word processor, spreadsheets)
- Using other resources (e.g. secretaries) to give you reminders or manage your diary if you are already working or if you have done summer jobs where this applied.

Example of an effective answer

I have always been efficient at organising my time so that I can fit in everything that I need to do within a busy day. During the past few years, I planned my revision carefully by looking at the amount of work that I would need to do in relation to the syllabus. I also allowed some time for outside activities, which enabled me to relax and be more efficient in my work.

Over the past few years, I have also become involved in organising a number of events within the school, all of which had tight deadlines that had to be met. This required careful planning and coordination with other members of the team. In order to meet the deadlines, I had regular discussions with my colleagues so that we could identify any potential problems and find solutions to minimise their impact.

Overall, I like to be punctual, to deliver my assignments on time and to complete my projects within a comfortable margin. To do so, I find it useful to keep a list of tasks that I need to do, either in my electronic diary or, in the case of a larger project, on a spreadsheet that I can update at regular intervals depending on developments. When I was responsible for social events at my school, I also made full use of the college's secretaries, who helped a great deal to ensure that everything ran smoothly and freed up some of my time when there were fires to be fought.

Note how each idea is backed up by a practical application and is not simply part of a long list.

9.13 How good are your organisational skills?

Organisational skills are closely linked to time management skills. As well as time management, they also include the ability to:

- Multitask
- Identify the right resources
- Plan effectively to get things done on time
- Prioritise
- Delegate/use the team effectively
- Adjust to unfolding events and reprioritise appropriately
- Stay focused on the task at hand.

Essentially, the examples will be very similar to those in Q 9.12.

Example of an effective answer

I have always enjoyed being busy and getting involved in several projects at the same time. For example, over the past year, I have studied for five A Levels, worked at weekends at a local charity shop and spent some time gathering some work experience in preparation for medical school. I have also kept up with my sporting activities and music commitments at the local music school. To achieve all this, I needed to be very organised and I feel that I have demonstrated good organisational skills.

In particular, it was essential that I planned my weeks reasonably early so that I could identify what I would need to prepare in anticipation. I allocated time slots in my schedule, which I would protect for my homework. I would also allocate proper time where I could relax and practise my hobbies. In terms of my academic work, I analysed on an ongoing basis how much work I would need to put in for the following week, taking account of planned examinations and assignments, and I arranged for suitable preparation time. I also arranged time with my friends so that we could revise some important topics together and go out afterwards. Being meticulous and organised has really helped me minimise stress by enabling me to achieve everything I needed to achieve; as a result I feel more than equipped to deal with the pressure of studying Medicine.

9.14 What are your hobbies?

The purpose of this question is to establish whether you have ways of re-laxing and whether you take an interest in things other than your work. There are several points that you should bear in mind when discussing your hobbies:

1. It is not a competition about who has got the most interesting hobby out of all the candidates, or who has got the weirdest hobby of all. You don't need to go cart-racing on Mount Everest every weekend to be an interesting candidate.

2. What really matters is the range of activities that you have, what they bring you and what you find interesting about them. You will get a place at medical school if you enjoy reading novels and cooking for friends, provided you are able to explain in a personal way why these things matter to you.

3. If most of your hobbies are solitary (such as reading and playing the piano), mention them but try to counterbalance them with other as-pects of your life that present you as a sociable person. It is not to say that you have to present yourself as a party animal, but a sociable human being would be good enough.

4. Don't try to lie about your hobbies or present, as hobbies, activities that are no more than just routine. For example, there is no point pre-tending that you like cooking if all you do is defrost pizzas, or that you enjoy photography if you only take holiday pictures of your boyfriend, girlfriend or dog. They might dig further into your answers and you run the risk of being found out.

5. You may extend the definition of "hobbies" to include other personal interests such as charity/voluntary work. It all helps to sell yourself!

Hobbies that you might mention

Music: Listening to opera, jazz, classical and ethnic music. Playing an instrument, singing, dancing. Be specific about what you do. Do you be-long to an orchestra or a choir or do you play at home? Did you achieve certain grades or have particular achievements you want to talk about?

Culture: Modern and classical arts, wine tasting and cooking, etc. Again be specific, but avoid mentioning wine tasting if you only do this on Friday evenings in a pub with your mates after five pints of beer! Cooking for friends and socialising can be an enjoyable thing to do.

Leisure: Travelling, stamp collecting, pottery, etc. Discuss where you travelled and what you enjoyed about it. Stamp collecting can be sociable if you belong to a club. If you do it by yourself, you can always go on about how you find it useful in teaching you patience, but you will need to counteract it with something more sociable to strike the right balance.

Sports: You can include team sports such as football, netball, hockey, etc. or individual sports such as skiing, cycling, walking and mountain climbing (most of these are sociable activities too).

Languages are good to demonstrate your commitment to learning, patience and a logical mind. Don't pretend you are an expert at Portuguese or Russian if you are not. You want to avoid being asked a question in Russian!

Example of an effective answer

I have many interests outside school. I enjoy team sports such as football, which I play regularly with my friends. It is a great way to de-stress at weekends after a hard week and I particularly enjoy the camaraderie that we have in the team.

I also love going to the opera and museums. I get very passionate about Mozart's operas and I regularly make the effort to go and watch them live at the Royal Opera House. I find that classical music enables me to clear my head, which in turn helps me be more focused when I need to be.

I noticed on the medical school website that there are hundreds of clubs on offer at the university and I am looking forward to trying new interests such as culinary clubs and dancing clubs. As you can see from my statement, I also learned French and German at GCSE level. I am hoping to consolidate my modern languages when I travel with my friends to Europe before starting medical school.

9.15 Tell me about a non-academic project in which you were involved

This question is a test of your drive and initiative. It asks for a specific project/example and therefore the STARR framework (see Section 6.3) will help you structure your answer. Through this question, you should sell yourself in terms of communication skills, teamwork and leadership as much as you can.

Non-academic projects can be for example:

- Sporting events such as football or netball tournaments (note that if you only played, you won't have much to talk about. Use this if you actually helped organised part of a project/event)
- Duke of Edinburgh Award Scheme
- Committee activities such as balls, charity events, cultural events
- Business projects you have set up.

Example of an effective answer

The non-academic project that I am most proud of is an online business that I recently set up and which is selling Italian gourmet products online.

I started by doing a lot of market research by talking to customers in shops, as well as friends and family, and I identified a gap in the market. One of the main problems was that I needed some capital in order to purchase some preliminary stock. My first approach was to contact several friends to help raise the £2000 that I needed as initial capital. I also involved my friends in the business and we worked hard as a team. Everyone contributed in accordance with their strengths. I delegated to one of them the task of setting up the website; others were better at negotiating and I involved them in purchasing the goods. Others helped with packing and shipping the items. Some members of my family are helping too when I am busy studying.

The business is expanding and we are also making a small profit. I am hoping the money will help to fund my gap year. Though I will need to pass on the reins to someone else when I am at medical school, I feel I have learnt a lot from that experience from attention to detail, to negotiation skills and multitasking.

9.16 How do you cope with stress?

This question frightens many candidates. Everyone thinks about mentioning a few hobbies, though few provide an explanation about why they enjoy those hobbies and their personal importance. Few actually go beyond the "hobbies" approach.

Why this question?

Stress is something that you will experience throughout medical school and your career as a doctor. You will be stressed for many reasons, including:

- Work overload and lack of resources
- Not being confident about your own abilities
- Making mistakes or fear of making them
- Working with difficult colleagues
- Unexpected events, both work and family related
- Unsocial hours
- Dealing with difficult patients
- Experiencing the harshest aspects of Medicine (seeing a patient die for the first time, seeing a sick child)
- Taking on difficult assignments such as breaking bad news to a patient
- Having to make a presentation in front of a large audience
- Having to find a good job that suits both your career and your social ambitions.

Stress is omnipresent and you simply cannot resolve every situation by playing football or playing the piano after work.

How to deal with stress

The way that you will deal with stress depends on its origin and the means available to you. You do not deal with long-term stress due to burning out in the same way that you deal with the immediate stress caused by a mistake that you have made.

Some of the ways of handling stress include:

- Making sure that you remain organised. (better planning and time management, prioritising tasks, taking tasks one at a time)
- Delegating tasks to others
- Taking breaks/time off
- Anticipating future problems and taking proactive steps to prevent them and minimise their impact
- Seeking advice from friends and colleagues. In Medicine you can also get independent advice from legal helplines often run by defence organisations, charities or even the GMC
- Reflecting on events and putting them into perspective
- Having a healthy lifestyle, hobbies and activities.

Example of an ineffective answer

I can cope with stressful situations such as exams. I always meditate and keep calm. I find this is very useful. I also play football and tennis to help me cope when I am stressed.

This example mentions a few basic ideas and does not present any information about how the candidate copes with stress other than by playing sport. This may be useful but not in all circumstances. The answer lacks depth and needs to be a bit more detailed in its approach (e.g. by quoting examples) and to encompass different aspects of stress.

Example of an effective answer

I always find that a bit of stress keeps me focused and gives me the adrenaline that I need to do well in my work. However, too much stress can potentially be destructive and I have learnt to deal with it in many different ways. I always try to keep calm, take a step back and evaluate the reasons behind the stress. Depending on the cause of the stress, I will react differently. For example, during my exam revisions, I had to deal with many topics at the same time, which put a lot of pressure on me time-wise. Having drawn a revision plan at the start, I took some time to review my plan halfway through to make sure that I could remain on target. I also found it important to take regular breaks as it helped me relax and ultimately helped me concentrate better. On a different note, a few years ago I had to deal with stress caused by illness in my family and I coped with that stress by talking to a few trusted friends about the situation, which helped a lot.

Generally speaking, I try to maintain a healthy lifestyle so that I am fully prepared to handle stressful situations whenever they arise. It also helps me to minimise my ability to get stressed in the first place. I try to eat healthily and I am involved in extra-curricular activities. I find running and playing football extremely helpful. They help to keep me calm and to release my frustrations. I also love listening to jazz; in particular, I find Miles Davis' music extremely calming. Finally, whenever I have had a difficult time, I find it useful to reflect on the situation and see how I can prevent something similar happening in future. I find that by doing this I grow more confident in being able to handle the unexpected.

Example of an effective answer

I deal with stress in very different ways depending on its causes at the time. For example this year, whilst I was taking my A Levels, I also had other responsibilities such as looking after my granddad when my parents went away, and having to deal with my little sister at the same time. That was stressful because it left me little time to revise properly. I dealt with it firstly by making a strict schedule that I could realistically adhere to and by sticking to it. Part of the stress in that situation was due to the fact that both my sister and my granddad expected me to give them more attention than I could afford and so I sat down with them to explain the situation and reassure them that I would be there for them without necessarily being able to spend every minute with them.

Another way in which I deal with stress is by making sure that I take regular breaks and have activities that I enjoy which help me relax. For example, over the past 2 years, I had to sacrifice football practice because it was taking too much of my time, but I made a point of keeping music practice in my schedule so that I always had something to look forward to. If I work particularly hard (for example during revision time) I found it helpful to allocate at least 30 minutes of my time to go for a walk to clear my head.

Overall I feel that I have managed to go through the last few years relatively untouched by stress. And I have every confidence that the way I structure my time and my life will equally help me go through the challenges that lay ahead at medical school.

9.17 How do you feel that your hobbies have contributed to or are relevant to your studies?

This question is very similar to Q.9.14: "What are your hobbies?" However, do not make the mistake of discussing your hobbies without addressing the second part of the question. You would be missing the point.

Whether you enjoy hockey or flower arranging is not really where the difference will be made at the interview (although unofficially some interviewers may have a subconscious preference for candidates who do sport or music).

One thing is certain: the marks will be higher for candidates who bring a personal reflection into their answer. If you have specific achievements (prizes, competitions), present them.

Example of an effective answer

I have always been interested in competitive sports such as rugby. I find competitive sports keep me focused and motivated. They also help me to push myself to the limit. I am now in a team that has won a number of cups. I hope to continue to pursue my passion for rugby when I am at medical school.

I find that rugby has contributed a lot to my studies. In the same way that a game is not won or lost until the last second of play, I always work hard and try my best in coursework to achieve my goals. I always stay focused and don't give up easily. Of course, rugby is also a team sport. I have made some brilliant friends at school through the club and I intend to continue to meet new friends in the same way. It contributed greatly to my studies in helping me appreciate the impact of good teamwork and good communication.

9.18 What are your main strengths? What attributes do you have that will make you a good doctor?

If you think about it, your mains strengths will need to be a close match to the requirements for a good medical student, which should be a close match for the attributes of a good doctor. These two questions are therefore extremely similar. The attributes that will make you a good doctor are varied, and would include:

- Fast learner. Always keen to learn more and improve
- Able to synthesise information
- Good manual dexterity (for surgeons or interventional physicians)
- Able to weigh information to make decisions
- Confident in decision making
- Humble. Able to reflect and recognise own limitations
- Focused on other people
- Good listener, empathic, able to build a rapport with people
- Caring and selfless
- Effective at conveying ideas in simple terms
- Good team player (see Q.9.5)
- Interested and proactive in teaching others
- Naturally curious
- Patient with others. Good motivator
- Good organisational skills (see Q.9.12)
- Able to handle stress effectively (see Q.9.16).
- Good leader (see Q.9.7)
- Approachable and supportive
- Friendly and sociable
- Objective
- Honest and trustworthy
- Personal and professional integrity
- Respects others.
- Constructive in dealing with problems and conflict.

The list is endless. Rather than present a very long list of attributes, try to concentrate on a few powerful concepts, which you can back up with examples. One important aspect of your answer is that it should be rigidly structured so that the interviewers are not presented with a self-gratifying ramble, but with information they can easily digest.

Example of an effective answer

I am conscientious and hard-working and, as a result, I consistently achieve high grades at school. I am also an enterprising person and I try to read a lot outside the curriculum in order to broaden my knowledge. In particular, I have read articles on scientific research such as the Human Genome Project and I am looking forward to doing some research when I become a doctor. It is also thanks to my entrepreneurial drive that I have succeeded in getting involved in very interesting work experience posts, both in a hospital and in the community.

Another one of my strengths is my communication skills. I am regarded by all my friends as someone who is very approachable and I feel that being a good listener is essential to building good relationships with people. I had the opportunity to test my listening skills and empathy when I did some work experience at a local hospice, where some of the patients told me that I had brightened up their day and helped them through simply by being there and showing some care and attention.

I am also a very organised person and I can work well under pressure. I have always enjoyed getting involved in a wide range of activities, whether they are academic projects or social activities. I also enjoy being part of groups where I can use my leadership skills. For example, I sit on the social committee at school. Because I have my hands in many projects at the same time, I have become very good at organising my time and also at using all the resources that I have to make sure that I can do everything on time and with a good quality outcome. I like working under pressure because it gives me a buzz and I feel that it helps me to stretch myself. Luckily, I also find time to fit in a couple of hobbies, which help me deal with all this stress and pressure. I am particularly keen on football, which I play regularly with my friends.

All these attributes will really help me during my career in Medicine and I am looking forward to developing them further during medical school and beyond.

There are three distinct paragraphs. Each paragraph deals with a separate idea and each idea is backed up by personal experience. Note how we have grouped together a number of ideas that are related (for example conscientious, hard-working and entrepreneurial in the first paragraph).

9.19	Why are you the best candidate today? Why should we take you on?

These are both the same question. Essentially, you are the best candidate because you fit all the requirements and more. This question is therefore similar to Q.9.18 about your main strengths. Make sure that you use a strong structure so that the information passes across to the interviewers effortlessly.

Example of an effective answer

I am sure all the candidates today are of a very high standard. However, I think I have many good qualities that make me stand out. Firstly, I have consistently demonstrated my commitment and devotion to Medicine. I have done a lot of work experience both for charities and shadowing consultants and GPs over the past 2 years. This has given me a really good understanding of what being a doctor is like.

Secondly, I have a good academic track record. I work hard and perform well in school. My head teacher has predicted straight 'A's in my A Levels. I am very encouraged by that. I am also a keen sportsman who understands the importance of teamwork. I also seize opportunities to enhance my leadership skills. For example, I have been involved in setting up various projects in my school and in organising football tournaments at my local school.

I am an approachable person who enjoys working with others and interacting with people at all levels. I have really learnt a lot about communication from my work experience and I feel that I have developed some good listening skills.

Finally, I am a dynamic, friendly, conscientious candidate and I believe that my motivation and inspiration will ensure a successful career in Medicine.

9.20 Give three adjectives that best describe you

Again a question very close to "What are your main strengths?" Your answer to this will very much depend on whether you want to cheat by discussing three concepts rather than giving three adjectives. For example, does "being a good communicator" fit the bill? Strictly speaking no because this is not an adjective, but they will probably let you get away with it.

If you want to "cheat" then you can answer the question in the same way that you addressed the "main strengths" question.

If you are more of a purist, then there are numerous adjectives that you can use, which will lead to similar answers:

Adaptable	Assertive	Approachable
Dynamic	Dedicated	Decisive
Friendly	Flexible	Dependable
Confident	Conscientious	Hard-working
Honest	Reliable	Trustworthy
Entrepreneurial	Focused	Motivated

Follow the models set out in the previous answers to highlight three adjectives that allow you to demonstrate wide-ranging qualities.

9.21 How would your friends describe you?
What would you like written in your obituary?

For those who don't know, an obituary is what people write in a newspaper when you have died and it therefore concentrates on your positive attributes and achievements. These two questions are therefore almost the same. They pose many problems to candidates when, in reality, they are no different to the previous questions about your strengths or about the adjectives that would best describe you.

Example of an effective answer

I have made friends in all the activities that I have undertaken and I think that they would describe me in a very positive light.

From a general perspective, people tend to see me as someone who is easy-going, friendly and approachable. I always try to make time for them if they want to have a chat. I am a good non-judgemental listener, which I think they appreciate.

I have also made friends at my basketball club, where I am the captain. People trust me to make good decisions and they would probably say that I am a very inclusive person who takes account of others' ideas and opinions but can also make clear decisions when needed. I think they would recognise that this has really helped the team achieve the success that it has had over the past 2 years. As well as being a good leader and motivator, they also regard me as a good team member, who enjoys socialising and has a good sense of humour.

Finally, I think that they would say that I am someone who is very honest and has a lot of integrity. I am the first to recognise when I have made a wrong decision, for example. Overall, they would agree that I am someone that they can depend on in all circumstances.

9.22 Do you have the personality that it takes to do Medicine?

If you ever considered answering "no" or "maybe" or "I don't know", you ought to think about an alternative career. There is only one possible answer to this question and it is "yes, of course".

Essentially it is asking: "Do you have what it takes to be a good doctor?" and you will therefore need to establish confidently that you are:

- Knowledgeable, competent, confident
- Keen to learn
- A good communicator and team player
- A good potential leader and well organised
- Able to work well under pressure
- Caring, sensitive, supportive, approachable
- Hard-working, enthusiastic, motivated, disciplined, conscientious
- Trustworthy, honest and have integrity

Example of an ineffective answer

The personalities that are needed to do Medicine are honesty, motivation, caring for patients and good discipline. I feel that I have all of these and I am ready to go into Medicine.

This answer does not work well for two reasons. It does not address a wide range of skills (what has happened to communication skills and teamwork?) and it does not really provide any personal backup to the claims made.

Effective answers
A good example would be any example derived as per Q.9.18, Q.9.19, Q.9.20 or Q.9.21, all of which are similar in nature to this question.

9.23 What skills have you gained in your current work, that are transferable to Medicine? (Question for graduates)

Wherever you are currently working, there are many skills that you may have used that are crucial in the day-to-day life of a doctor and therefore that are directly transferable. These skills include your ability to:

- Listen effectively and identify client needs
- Explain complex issues in a simple language
- Organise complex information, summarise and present it
- Identify resources needed to help you reach your goals
- Seek expert advice when required
- Manage third parties
- Negotiate with third parties
- Use your initiative to resolve complex problems
- Identify areas of change and implement corresponding solutions
- Work independently and as part of a team
- Lead a group of people
- Influence others to your point of view
- Work to tight deadlines
- Deal with conflicting demands on your time and on your resources
- Deal with stress
- Handle conflict
- Manage difficult colleagues or clients
- Identify areas for development
- Provide good customer service, beyond requirements
- Develop your own knowledge and skills, and drive your own career.

You simply need to identify a handful of skills that you feel are characteristic of your current position and to present them following the same technique as set out in the previous questions. You should explain in what context you have developed those skills and how relevant they will be to you in Medicine.

See Q.9.18 to Q.9.21 for possible models of answers.

9.24 Do you work better by yourself or as part of a team?

This is a trick question and many candidates, in their eagerness to appear sociable, come out with "As part of a team of course". Essentially, the short answer is: both. Of course, as a doctor it is crucial that you are able to work well as part of a team. However, there will also be many opportunities where you will need to make decisions by yourself, or where others will simply expect you to deliver results without necessarily relying on other team members at all times. In other words, you should also be able to demonstrate that you can get on with things and take the initiative.

Working by yourself does not mean that you are antisocial. It can also mean that you are dependable and can take responsibility to get on with your work. In your answer, you simply need to describe both sides, give examples from your experience and explain how this relates to Medicine.

Example of an effective answer

I can work well both as part of a team and on my own. In the past I have been part of different types of teams. For example, I play football and, during the summer, I spent time working as a sales assistant. I have always communicated well with my colleagues and been very supportive. I have always been proactive in contributing in team meetings, in involving others in my work when needed and in showing willingness to help out.

At the same time, I can also take responsibility for my work and I am able to deliver results by myself when expected. This is not to say that I work totally independently, but I am able to get on with my work so that I can report back to my team at a later stage. For example, when I was on the social committee at my school, being in charge of the budget for my team, there were times when I needed to interact with my colleagues and other times when I simply needed to spend some time on my own so that I could concentrate on the complexity of the problem and deliver a financial solution that made sense in view of all the input that I had received during the consultation process.

The same applies to Medicine. Work is agreed as a team and you can draw on the team's resources to help resolve any issues. But there comes a stage where you also have to work independently in order to get the work done.

9.25 What is your main weakness?

This is a question that sends shivers down everyone's spine all the way to consultant interviews! Ask anyone how best to address this question and everyone will give you a different answer, telling you that their way is best because one of their friends got into medical school by giving that answer.

Some people got into medical school by saying that they didn't have any weakness and some people got rejected for saying the same thing. Some people got accepted by saying that they were perfectionists and others got rejected because that answer was too corny. Some people even got into medical school by saying that their main weakness was that they liked chocolate ice cream too much.

The truth is that any answer should be viewed in its context, in relation to the person who delivers it, the people who receive it, their sense of humour, what they would themselves have said at an interview, etc. It is extremely difficult to give advice to derive an answer that will guarantee success; nevertheless, there are answers that are safer than others and we seek to explain below how we feel the question should be approached.

The corny and the unwise answers

Some answers are definitely unwise or very risky:

- "I don't have any weakness" – the aim of this question is really to establish whether you are aware of your negative traits and how you are addressing them. Not having any weaknesses will not make you a better human being or a better doctor. In fact, it may present you as someone who is arrogant and refuses to admit that there are aspects that you could improve.

- "I am not very good at anatomy" or any other topic – not wise. If you are not good at a topic that you have chosen, and which is highly relevant for Medicine, that will be the end of the day for you.

- "I am disorganised" – there are some fundamental requirements for Medicine that you should not consider highlighting as a weakness. Doctors should be organised, keep their cool under pressure, be able to handle stress, etc. If you are disorganised, you will find it difficult to cope. Personal organisation is something that is difficult to change and therefore you would not really be selling anything positive as part of your answer.

- "My handwriting is not very legible" – same as above. Clear and legible handwriting is crucial to ensure accuracy of the notes and the safety of patients (imagine the consequences of a nurse misunderstanding your dosages) and is tested on recruitment all the way to consultant level. If your handwriting is bad, it will never really improve and it may go against you.

- "I eat too much chocolate" – great! We have really learnt a lot about you here. You never know; it has been known to work.

- "I am a perfectionist" – the problem with this weakness is that this answer is probably given by 50% of candidates and therefore you will not go very far with it. So, although the weakness by itself is perfectly fine to mention, it is the wording that causes a problem by being overused. Also, being a perfectionist can have different meanings and, if you really want to develop this concept, you would need to be a lot more specific. More later ...

- "I can't say 'no' to people" – the problem is the same as for the "perfectionist" answer. The concept suffers from overuse and is not developed enough to have any impact. More later too ...

Presenting a strength as a weakness

This is a technique often used by candidates and, in principle, it is probably the best way to handle the question. For example, having high expectations can be a strength because it means you are striving for quality. But it can also be a weakness because it could make relationships difficult with others at times.

Although many candidates are on the right track with this approach, they ruin their chances by taking a light-hearted approach to the question. In an effort to get rid of it as soon as possible because it feels uncomfortable, they become evasive and lose the personal touch that the question calls for. For example, "I have a tendency to focus too much on detail and, although this can be a good thing, it can also be a weakness" may be a good concept in principle but it feels really impersonal and empty of any really meaningful content.

Suggested approach

Our suggestion is to take an approach that is both explanatory and personal.

The first thing to recognise is that most weaknesses are actually strengths that have been pushed too far and which, under some circumstances, have become a real weakness. Therefore, rather than pretending that your weakness is really a strength (which may give the impression that you are trying to fob off the interviewers), you can be a lot more accurate by describing a real strength that you have which is sometimes becoming a weakness.

Secondly, you must be descriptive and use your experience to back up everything you say. This is the only way that you can make a real impact on your interviewers. Describe the strength and why it is a strength. Explain how it can become a weakness and how this has affected you in the past. If you can, give a concrete example.

Thirdly, describe how you react to this weakness, how you identify it, and what you are doing to remedy it. Again, be practical.

Worked examples

The answer "I am a perfectionist" is only cheesy because the wording has become a common phrase at interviews and because candidates do not often bother to explain what they mean by it. Being a perfectionist can mean many things. It can mean that you have high expectations of others. It can also mean that you do not always see the larger picture and pay too much attention to small detail, particularly when you become stressed.

Example of an effective answer (high expectations of others)

I am someone who is constantly striving to achieve the best and I have high expectations of myself as well as others. On one hand it can help me achieve a lot in my work, but there are occasions where it can become an issue, especially if my own expectations do not necessarily match those of others. I can remember one particular occasion where I was part of a group organising a big fund-raising event. My role consisted of organising the catering and I was keen to achieve the best possible quality for the budget available. As a result, I placed a lot of conditions on the caterers and consequently most pulled out of the bidding process. This forced me to review my criteria, which lost us 2 days in the organisation of the event.

Ultimately, I was able to recognise where I had gone wrong and worked hard to rebuild contact with the caterers to make the event a success. Part of the issue was that I had only listened to part of the advice that some of the caterers had given me. I learnt a lot from this experience. In particular, I am a lot more aware of the times when I can be too demanding and have learnt to think more carefully before I issue instructions and requests to others. It has also taught me to be more open to suggestions from everyone rather than just a few selected people. In this particular case, although I had taken account of my colleagues' suggestions, I had not fully taken on board the caterers' comments. In many ways, this is something that I can improve further through experience and exposure to different situations and I feel that I have already improved quite a lot in that respect.

Note that in this answer we have not mentioned anywhere the word "perfectionist". Instead we have defined one of its meanings more accurately.

We have also illustrated the weakness through an example, which gives it more realism and helps the interviewers de-dramatise the weakness and understand it in a real-life context. In turn, this enables you to explain how you cope with the weakness from a practical point of view, which helps personalise the answer.

Note also how the example presents a personal reflection towards the end, explaining what the candidate has learnt from the situation and how he is working on improving.

Example of an effective answer (too much attention to detail)

My main weakness is perhaps that I sometimes pay a little too much attention to detail and, as a result, I can spend more time than I really should on matters that do not necessarily have that much of an impact on the overall result. For example, I spent many hours writing and correcting the personal statement that I have submitted for this university application. It has obviously done the trick because I am sitting here today but I am fairly sure that I could have achieved the same result by spending a third less time on it. I guess that fundamentally it is about wanting to do my very best but that there has to be a trade-off somewhere between the time spent and the result achieved.

I feel that this is something that I am getting better at, partly by observing the way my friends work and discussing this issue with them. I am also improving as I gain more confidence in myself and in my capabilities.

"I can't say 'no'"

"I can't say 'no'" is also a common answer, which makes it ineffective. Again, the problem is not so much with the concept behind it – this is a good weakness to mention – but more with the phraseology.

It can actually mean different things. On the positive side, it can mean that you are a good team player, willing to get involved and to please others. It could also mean that you are ambitious and are keen to get involved in many activities. Identify the messages that you are trying to put across and make them explicit.

On the negative side, it can lead to overload of work, stress, people taking advantage of you, less time for your family, etc.

With regard to what can be done to resolve the problem, people often state that they have learnt to say "no". You must be careful not to go the other way by presenting yourself as someone who is no longer a team player. The answer is not always to start saying no to others, but for you to become more realistic about what you have the time to do, to work with others to make them understand your situation, to make sure that you understand their situation and for both of you to come to an agreement. You must learn to be more in control and maybe to be a bit more assertive.

Putting all this together and incorporating an example would give:

I am someone who is ambitious and I like getting involved in numerous projects in order to achieve a lot and develop new skills. However, sometimes it can get a little too much to deal with.

For example, over the past 12 months, I studied for five A Levels, I got involved in running a youth club on Wednesday evenings, I played football with young kids at weekends, I learnt to drive and spent a lot of time gaining work experience in the evening at the local hospice and at a GP surgery on Fridays. I got involved in some of these social activities because people were asking me to get involved and I did not want to disappoint them. However, in hindsight, I realise that it placed me in a difficult situation where I had rather a lot to handle all at once, which was sometimes quite stressful.

This is an issue that has occasionally arisen in the past and I feel that I am getting better at recognising what I can realistically get involved in and what I can't. I have learnt to manage people's expectations by being honest with them about my workload but also by trying to see how I might be able to find a solution without being directly involved every time.

This has eased up the pressure on my time and I now feel much more confident in dealing with these requests.

Other possible weaknesses that you can mention

Ultimately, there are many weaknesses that you can discuss and which, if illustrated by the right example, are perfectly palatable at an interview. Possible weaknesses include:

- Taking criticism too personally – this is a perfectly normal reaction and provided that you explain how you are changing in that respect by seeing criticism as a way to improve then you will be fine.

- Being over-empathic. Many people go into Medicine because they are caring and empathic. But these attributes, which are real strengths, can become weaknesses when you deal with very ill patients to whom you might get attached. You have to learn to harden your skin and this will come through experience.

- Being direct with people. This is a good attribute as people know exactly what you mean and it avoids confusion. However, there are situations where tact is required; and so you must also explain that you are learning through experience to adopt a more mellow approach when the situation calls for it.

9.26 If you could change two things about yourself, what would they be?

This is also a weakness-type question, but this time they are asking for two! People are often reluctant to talk about their weaknesses, understandably so. However, if prepared properly, these answers can make a real difference compared to other candidates who may come up with a bland answer. Remember that discussing your weaknesses shows a good personal insight and a willingness to improve. Use these questions to your advantage. Most of your success will depend on how confident you are in delivering your answer as much as on its content. You can inspire yourself with the previous question to get some ideas about what you can say.

Example of an effective answer

One thing I would like to change about myself is learning not to take on too much at the same time. I am always eager to get involved in various projects. For example, last year, as well as having to study for five A Levels, I was working weekends at a local charity shop, did some coaching for kids who wanted to play football and took piano lessons. Although I managed to cram everything in, it could sometimes prove quite stressful. Part of the issue was that I did not want to let anyone down when they asked me if I wanted to get involved, so I guess it might just be a case of being a bit more self-confident and assertive when needed.

Another thing that I would like to change about myself is to learn to live more healthily. When I am busy I don't tend to have such a healthy diet and I tend to neglect my usual exercise regime. It is something that I have noticed over the past year and that I will need to address as soon as I get into medical school. I guess that having a number of sport clubs on-site will be a great help in that regard.

9.27 Who has had a major influence on you as a person?

This question is not so much about who as it is about why. Ultimately, it does not really matter if the person who influenced you most was your father, your older brother, a teacher, the local priest or Lord Nelson. What really matters is how they inspired you and the qualities that they demonstrated that you found attractive. This question is therefore about you, not them. Consequently, in your answer you will need to detail what qualities you found inspiring in that person and how you incorporated those qualities within your own life.

The qualities that you may wish to demonstrate through your answer could be:

Competent	Good motivator	Good listener
Confident	Inspirational	Good teacher
Assertive	Approachable	Inclusive
Fair	Supportive	Committed
Decisive	Caring	Dedicated
Conscientious	Patient	Friendly
Hard-working	Enthusiastic	Careful
Optimistic	Empathic	

Try to use a broad combination of three/four of the above or others you may find relevant and develop each one in turn. Note that the person in question does not have to be a doctor. There are inspiring people outside Medicine too!

Example of an ineffective answer

My father has been a major influence in my life. He is hard-working and supports my brothers and me through school. I hope I can become a good GP to make him proud.

There is nothing wrong with mentioning the father and the GP ambition. But the answer lacks detail about the qualities that the father has or had.

Example of an effective answer

One of the people who had a major influence on my life and whom I respected greatly was my uncle, who worked as a marketing director in a local engineering firm. He was someone who always saw life from a positive point of view, despite the problems that he faced at the time in terms of job uncertainty. I used to go with him to see clients during my school holidays and I observed him deal with them in many different ways. He was always very attentive to his clients, trying to understand what they really wanted so that he could deliver the best to them. Whenever clients had a complaint, he always treated them with respect and took a proactive attitude in resolving the problems that they had encountered.

At home, he was also always a good family man, very attentive to his family and never afraid of going out of his way to help out. When I was 10 years old, I lost a good friend in a car crash and my uncle was very supportive in trying to help me get over it. Sometimes he did not do much else than simply sit with me and listen to me, but I found this to be a great help.

Overall, he was a very caring man dedicated to both his family and his work. He also enjoyed life to the full and knew how to have a good time to relax and take a break from his worries. This is how he inspired me, and in many ways I am aspiring to develop the same balance in life that he had.

Note how the answer deals with a few points only, which are backed up with a few personal examples. An effective answer does not have to list 20 qualities. Go for quality rather than quantity. It will help you make your point more effectively and will enable you to come across as more personal and more enthusiastic too.

9.28   What makes a good teacher?

Teaching is an essential activity in a doctor's life. Just as you have been taught by other doctors, you will be expected to teach others too. A good way of formulating your ideas is as follows:

Knowledge: a good teacher has a thorough understanding of his subject. This enables him to be credible with his students by appearing competent. With a strong knowledge, a teacher is also able to address any issues or questions that students may have.

Communication skills: a good teacher should be able to take advanced information and to translate it into a language that is easily understood by his audience. A bad teacher would make the same information confusing. A good teacher is also able to choose teaching methods that are appropriate to the audience and to the topic being discussed.

Generating interest: the best teachers will encourage students to learn by generating in his students an interest in the topic. A bad teacher will ensure that students are interested by generating a fear of failure (e.g. "if you do not know this, you will fail your exams"). In order to generate interest, a good teacher will need to be passionate himself about the topic.

Respect: a good teacher must be respected by his students. To achieve this, he must build credibility by being thoroughly prepared for teaching sessions, by being fair in his assessment of the students, by making himself available to discuss issues that students will raise during or after the session and, generally speaking, by ensuring that he provides the best quality to his students at all times.

Approachable and supportive: a good teacher is someone who looks after his students, is available to answer questions, is prepared to stretch the strong students and support those who struggle.

When you answer such a generic question, be careful not to confine yourself to answering the question in its narrowest interpretation. Make sure you give examples of good behaviours demonstrated by some of your teachers. You can also give examples of situations where you have demonstrated those qualities.

9.29 Tell us about your best/worst teacher?

Again this is a question about someone who inspired you (or did not), but this time they are imposing the context. It has to be a teacher. It does not matter who this teacher was; what matters is why they were good or bad. Many candidates waste their time with a single-line answer of the type "My best teacher was Mr Smith last year". Good for them, but not that interesting if there is no explanation as to why they were good.

Example of an effective answer (best teacher)

My best teacher is Mr Jones, my biology teacher for the past 2 years. He is someone that I really found inspiring for many reasons. First, he has an absolute passion for his subject and this really comes across in the way he teaches. He is clear in his explanations, he makes sure that we have understood the main messages before the end of the class, he makes his lesson fun by introducing variety and experiments, and he also makes sure that everyone in the class is involved by making his sessions interactive. This creates a really good environment and has actually helped the class gel together more.

Also, he is very good natured and he has never hesitated in staying beyond hours to help me understand a particular aspect on which I wanted more details. Whenever I made mistakes in answering a question or in an assignment, he was never over-critical but, on the contrary, he tried to find different ways of explaining the concept so that I could grasp it more easily.

And finally, he is also someone who I could approach easily if there were issues that I need to discuss, even if they related to matters outside biology. He is very caring and I am sure that he has played an important role in helping me decide to become a doctor.

Example of an effective answer (worst teacher)

My worst teacher was probably my arts teacher last year. She simply could not understand why everyone could not be good at arts and she insisted on giving attention only to those who were good at it. This meant that 90% of the class were effectively neglected and saw the arts classes as a chore.

She also made sarcastic comments about some students' work, including mine, and it was hard to take it in good humour and ignore the humiliation that came with it. In my mind a good teacher is someone who is able to adapt to his students and should certainly be someone who encourages those who are not at the top. He should also be open-minded, especially in a discipline as subjective as arts.

Teaching is something that I enjoy doing myself and in fact I coach 10-year-old kids at football on Wednesdays. Unlike this arts teacher, I believe in encouraging people and I think I have been able to do this successfully so far.

Note how the answer reversed the situation by explaining in the first instance why the teacher was bad and by using this as an opportunity to explain what makes a good teacher. Note also the personal conclusion.

9.30 Describe a time when you made a life-changing decision

This is a question asking for an example. Therefore you should use the STARR strategy (see Section 6.3) to answer this question. Outline the context, explain what you did, how you did it and why, and conclude by describing the outcome and what you learnt from the situation. This question is not just about the decision in itself. For example, if you simply said: "The life-changing decision I made was to decide to become a doctor", you will not provide any real information. As part of your answer you will need to describe the thinking process behind that decision and the risks that you were taking. This is really about how you approach a problem which does not have an obvious solution and which has important consequences. Can you see a parallel with Medicine here?

Example of an effective answer (dramatic)

About 5 years ago, my grandmother was placed into a home where she could be cared for in better conditions than at home. One evening we were called at home because she had suffered a heart attack and they had managed to resuscitate her. The doctor wanted to discuss "Do not resuscitate orders" with us because she was at risk of a relapse and was not able to make decisions.

They were in favour of issuing an order and my parents and I went to the hospital to discuss things through with the doctor. This gave rise to a big debate in the family and I was split between the grief of having to let my grandmother die and the rational thought that she would probably be more at peace and suffering less if we let her die. This was particularly important to me because I was very close to her.

Despite my personal grief, I told my parents that I felt that the doctors were best placed to make the decision and that she should not be resuscitated.

My grandmother subsequently died and I have often wondered what would have happened if we had decided to fight the decision. However, I am contented by the fact that she had lived a full life and died with dignity.

Another example of an effective answer (less dramatic)

Throughout my school years, I have been equally good at classic subjects such as English, history and economics as I have been in subjects such as physics, chemistry and biology. As a result, at one point, I was attracted to careers in both Law and Medicine, two specialties which dealt with making a difference to people, albeit in very different ways. That meant having to make a difficult choice when it came to my A Levels as the choice would then dictate which career I would embark upon.

In the first instance I had some informal chats with my family and friends. But, more importantly, I organised shadowing and work experience in both subjects so that I could make a more informed decision. That led me to conclude that, although I enjoyed the excitement of the legal process, the way in which arguments are put together and the good that could come out of it, in fact I could find those same features within Medicine as well albeit in a different context. Medicine also had the advantage that, aside from enabling me to use my communication skills and a methodical approach to problem solving, it also had a scientific side which is lacking in law.

I therefore drew the conclusion that Medicine was the right choice and here I am!

Note how the answers describe the thinking process and do not simply state the type of decision that was made. The second answer has the advantage of emphasising why the candidate chose Medicine, which can't hurt.

What if you have not had a life-changing event?

There is no point in making one up; it will be obvious from the lack of detail in your answer. You could rephrase the question by starting with "I can't say I have had a life-changing event in my life but I have certainly made some important decisions." And then go on to describe one of them.

9.31 What is your greatest achievement?

This is a very broad question, which could attract all kinds of answers. This could be an academic or a personal achievement, linked either to a single event or a lifelong achievement.

Examples include:

- Specific grades that you achieved or prizes that you won
- Ambitions that you have fulfilled through hard work or despite adverse conditions
- Projects in which you were involved, where you made a difference
- Success in anything that was competitive (the higher the competition, the better).

Whatever you mention, it must be a real achievement and you must describe what makes it an achievement. For example:

- Passing your driving test is not really an achievement unless you did it when you were busy and had little time for lessons, or unless you passed it after having spent weeks in plaster.
- Getting a 98% mark for your assignments is not an achievement if everyone else got 99%. Where do your marks place you?
- Speaking four languages is not an achievement if all you can say is "Bonjour", "Buongiorno", "Una cerveza por favor", "Sauerkraut, bitte". If, however, you can demonstrate you have taken it to an exceptional level then that would be an achievement.

Finally, you must explain what you did to gain this achievement (selling a few important leadership, team playing, initiative and communication skills in the process) and explain what it means to you.

Example of an effective answer

One of my greatest achievements was to organise fund-raising activities in favour of a local child who needed to go to the US for a life-saving operation. I enlisted the help of two friends and we set out to organise a number of activities over the course of the year.

We worked hard together to plan all the events. We split up the tasks according to our strengths and preferences. I organised regular meetings with my friends so that we could touch base and deal with any problems. I also asked for advice from other people who had organised similar events before and went out in the field to find companies who would be willing to offer sponsorship in return for advertisements during the events.

We raised over £5,000 and the child could go to the USA for the operation. I was proud of what we had achieved as a group and of the tenacity and enterprise that I demonstrated to achieve such a great result.

Another example of an effective answer

I have always been a keen sportsman and have always seen sport as a means to test my ability to surpass myself. Since I was a child I have been successful in several local competitions, winning a few medals on the way.

Last year, I was given a chance to enter a national fencing competition. Fencing is one of my favourite sports because it is about technique and precision rather than strength and the competitive atmosphere is often more friendly than in other sports. Out of 30 people selected for the competition, I came third. I felt it was amazing to have been selected for a national event through the hard work that I had put in at a local level, but coming third gave me a real sense of achievement. I had to work hard to achieve this, including attending extra training sessions; no mean feat in view of the fact I had to revise for my exams at the same time. But all my hard work paid off and I managed to get good grades in my exams too.

9.32 What are you most proud of?

This question is very similar to the previous question. In fact, you could actually give the same answer, since you will obviously be proud of any of your achievements.

However, you may also consider the question in a slightly broader sense, as you could also be proud of particular skills that you may have acquired. For example, you may be proud of the way in which you developed good communication skills or good organisation skills through a variety of means or events. You may also be proud of the fact that whenever you faced difficulties you always kept your spirits up and worked hard to find a solution to your problems. Nevertheless, if you choose this approach, you will need to back up your claims with examples and will need to discuss actual achievements, which takes us back, again, to the previous question.

Example of an effective answer

I am particularly proud of the organisation and time management skills that I have developed over the years. I am particularly proud of the success of the final year's sports day that I organised.

I was in charge of the whole programme. I enlisted the help of some friends to whom I delegated some important tasks to help me set up the sports activities, fund-raising programmes, prizes and also the guest invitations. I had discussions with everyone involved so that we could set realistic targets and prioritise the work accordingly. I also organised regular meetings so that we could share ideas and resolve any outstanding issues. Through good organisational skills, teamwork and a lot of effort, we produced a successful event that we were all proud of.

9.33 How do you cope with criticism?

Through this question, the interviewers want to test that you have an open approach and that you are keen to learn and to improve. They also want to know that you can take proactive action to resolve problems and that you are able to communicate effectively in a context where you may be placed on the defensive. This is the message that you need to communicate through your answer. If you can, give examples to illustrate the points that you are making.

Example of an effective answer

I guess that depends on the type of criticism that I face.

I have been in many situations where people have made some valuable observations which gave me cause to reflect on my own approach. For example, my parents told me off recently for revising too much and not focusing on the conversation during dinner. A few months ago one of my teachers told me that I had missed an important point in one of my presentations. In situations such as these, I try not to take things personally. I gracefully accept that I have made a mistake and try to improve for next time.

I have also been in situations where I felt I was unjustly criticised, or criticised by people who were doing it in a nasty or non-constructive manner. For example, during a recent football match, I missed a penalty and we lost the match. Some of my team members subsequently placed the entire blame on me, when it was quite clear that if they had been scoring goals themselves we may actually have won. In situations like these, it is tempting to rise to the bait and argue back (and to be honest, sometimes I do albeit trying to remain diplomatic); but on the whole I tend to take on board what is being said, allow myself time to calm down and then decide whether there are any points of value in their comments or whether there is nothing I can do about it. One thing I have learnt recently is that, even if you think there no validity to a particular criticism aimed at you, those who criticise always feel that they are in the right. In some cases the criticism can come across as harsh because they aren't always able to word it nicely, but it doesn't mean that they are necessarily wrong. That's why, on the whole, I try to remain open-minded.

9.34 How do you cope with conflict?

In a conflict question, the interviewers will be testing your ability to listen, be tactful and diplomatic and seek a constructive solution. Again, make sure you give examples to illustrate your points.

Example of an effective answer

As captain of the hockey team, I occasionally have to deal with conflicts between team members. These occur for various reasons ranging from a disagreement over tactics that we may use in a forthcoming game to conflict between two members who have become annoyed with each other following someone's mistake during a match. We have also had conflict between people who were fighting to be selected for the same position. My approach has always been to find the best way to resolve the issue as quickly as possible while making sure that I could preserve the team spirit. The team has grown stronger as a result. My first approach is to identify where the tension lies and to discuss the issue separately with each protagonist. This usually enables me to get a lot of information about how everyone feels and avoids direct confrontation. If I feel that I need to do so, then I might also ask for advice from other team members who may have ideas to resolve the problem, though I am sometimes reluctant to involve too many people at one time. I try to remain as flexible and fair as possible and I also try hard to make the two parties work on a way forward rather than attempting to impose my own point of view. I think that, ultimately, it is crucial to try to obtain a win-win outcome or at least a face-saving outcome and this is what I aim to achieve through discussion and negotiation. Of course, my main preoccupation is really to anticipate and prevent possible conflict so I work hard to ensure that the team members get on well together. When conflict does occur, having a close team also helps a lot in ensuring a quick resolution.

Other conflict situations that you can discuss include having to deal with a difficult person in one of your summer jobs. For example, if you had to discuss how you dealt with a difficult customer at the service desk, you could detail how you made sure that you let them express their opinion to allow them to vent their anger and to get all the facts. You could talk about how you made sure that you remained calm and identified another colleague who had the right knowledge and skills to help you out, etc.

9.35	**Give an example of a situation where you held an opinion but had to change your view**

This question is about a range of skills, including personal integrity, team playing, honesty and willingness to learn. Since it is a question asking for an example, you will need to use the STARR approach (see Section 6.3), describing first the situation and the opinion that you had formed. Secondly, you will need to outline what happened that made you change your mind, explaining in detail the thinking process that you went through and how you felt about the situation at the time. Finally, explain how the situation ended, emphasising what you learnt about it and yourself at the time.

Example of an effective answer

On my way to school, I have to cross an area of my town where a lot of homeless people sleep and it can sometimes feel a little unsafe if you are on your own. I had the preconception that homeless people were people who had little initiative and were simply happy living off other people's money. My beliefs were fuelled to some extent by anecdotal evidence on TV or in newspapers that some homeless people could earn a lot of money simply by begging.

Discussing the topic with one of my friends, he mentioned that he knew someone who had held a highly paid job and had ended up homeless following a bitter divorce from his wife. His comment puzzled me and I wondered whether I had simply misunderstood their situation from the beginning. We discussed the matter further and eventually decided to have a chat with some of the people that we saw every day on the pavement. There, we found an amazing mix of people, each with their own sad story but with a background and a level of education that was sometimes astonishing.

Following that episode, my friend and I started working at a local shelter one day per week and carried on chatting to our new friends on occasions. This really showed me how easy it can be to be prejudiced and how we must make sure that we know all the facts before passing judgement.

9.36 What is the worst mistake that you have made?

Like any negative question, you should not regard it as an attempt to trick you into saying something horrible, but instead as an opportunity for you to explain how you react in adverse circumstances. This includes your ability to show integrity throughout your behaviour.

In order to make the answer interesting, it will need to be an event where you learnt a valuable lesson. If the worst mistake that you have made is to choose rope climbing instead of athletics at school, there won't be much to talk about. On the other hand, try to strike the right balance by not choosing an example with consequences that can be regarded as extreme. They won't forgive you for having put your neighbour's cat in the microwave for the sake of scientific experimentation.

Doctors are human and make mistakes. You need to get over it. What really matters is that, when you make a mistake, you are able to:

- Spot it and own up to it (insight, honesty)
- Take immediate steps to correct it (initiative)
- Involve the right people to advise and help out (teamwork and communication)
- Apologise accordingly (honesty, communication)
- Analyse the situation to identify what went wrong and draw lessons from it (willingness to improve)
- Apply the lessons learnt to other similar situations
- Ensure others do not make the same mistake.

If you can discuss as many of the above points as possible, your answer will be complete.

Example of an effective answer

I would say that my worst mistake is possibly a wrong decision that I made during a Duke of Edinburgh expedition which went wrong as a result of it. I was the team member who was responsible for the equipment for directions. The mistake was to forget to charge the battery of the equipment before the event.

When we were in the forest, the equipment failed. At first I felt that something was not quite right but I was fairly confident that we would be able to reach our destination so I did not mention it to the others straight away. As we got lost further inside the forest, reality dawned on me and I felt increasingly uncomfortable at the idea of having to face my angry team mates' reaction. I mentioned tactfully to the team leader that I may have made a mistake and that we needed to stop to discuss the situation before it became potentially more difficult to resolve. I apologised to my team mates for having forgotten to check the equipment thoroughly and explained that we had got lost as a result. I emphasised that I took full responsibility for our position and that I would work hard to put us back on track, but that I also needed their assistance to achieve this. At first, some of the team members were angry but, after a while, we all pulled together and had a fruitful discussion about what our next steps should be. Eventually, and only an hour late, we made it to our destination. The next day, this became an endless topic for jokes and, in the end, the incident had actually made us closer as a team for having shared this experience.

I learnt quite a lot from the incident, and particularly how important it is to own up to your mistakes quickly so that they can be resolved as soon as possible. This also showed me how important it is to apologise and communicate effectively as it helps bring people on board. Finally, it gave me an opportunity to witness first hand how forgiving friends can be and that honesty is always the best policy.

Note the use of the word "possibly" at the beginning, which helps in softening the impact of what is coming afterwards (i.e. you pretend that you do not remember well at the beginning, so it can't be that bad). It all helps!

9.37 Tell us about an interesting book that you have read or film that you have seen

This question is fairly common and, contrary to appearance, it is not primarily designed to detect whether you have weird or eclectic tastes. No one will mind if you prefer watching horror movies instead of *The Little House on the Prairie* or if you prefer light-hearted comedies to books on social issues. What really matters is that there is something that interests you in the first place and that you are able to discuss why you enjoyed it.

Since you are only required to speak about one book or one film, it may be a good idea to place that book or film into the context of everything else that you enjoy reading or watching.

Book or film?

Generally speaking, it is a safer bet to discuss a book than a film because:

- The success of a film does not rest entirely on the story line but also very much on the actors that it contains. If the interviewers happen to dislike the main actor or if the storyline was weak, you may struggle to make any impact.

- Books are more neutral in their approach and people do not tend to have such strong preconceived ideas about them. In addition they represent a greater effort from your part (it takes longer to read a book than to watch a film with the same story) and this may subconsciously go in your favour.

Which one should you choose?

The choice of a good book or film is always difficult. You should select a book or film that you have really enjoyed so that you can talk about it in a passionate way. Each type of book or film can help you raise different issues. For example:

- **Biographies** are an ideal platform to discuss social issues, how success can be reached and how to overcome hurdles, how someone may have inspired you, etc. (assuming you read Mandela's or Gandhi's biography and not Donald Duck's).

- **Novels** are a good platform to raise social issues, stories about good and bad communication, resilience, power, etc., all of which can then be discussed in a generalised fashion. Again you would need to select a novel that would place you in a positive light to start with (e.g. you might think about avoiding mentioning Barbara Cartland).

- **Thrillers/Crime novels** are a good tool to talk about the power of analysis and deduction, together with the satisfaction of following a hero through the process. Crime novels are also a good platform to reflect on teamwork, leadership and communication.

- **Comedies** can be mentioned although you would need to make sure that you can derive more out of them than a simple indescribable personal enjoyment.

Whatever you wish to choose, ensure that you do not limit yourself to quoting a title and an author. Go into some depth about what you gained from the film or the book.

Example of an effective answer

One of the books that I found interesting recently is *The Da Vinci Code* by Dan Brown. Looking beyond the controversy that the book created, I found that it was thoroughly entertaining as it had a good pace and an enjoyable plot, full of intrigue. Although I never felt that it was written in the best possible prose, I thought that Dan Brown did very well in keeping the reader's imagination despite the complexity of the scenario. One of the other aspects that I enjoyed about the book is the manner in which it interprets the history of arts and the manner in which it portrays Michelangelo's work.

Generally speaking, I enjoy reading all sorts of books ranging from historical novels to biographies and thrillers. I try to read two or three good books per month. I find reading very soothing and I feel that it complements well the other activities that I do, such as sport and music, to help me relax when I have been exposed to pressure and stress.

Note how the description steers clear of the controversies surrounding the book and presents a generic critique of the content of the book from a personal perspective. Also, the answer highlights a few features of the book from your point of view but does not go into a massive amount of detail (you don't want to bore the interviewers). If they want to know more, they can ask; it will give you an opportunity to take the interview to the level of a discussion rather than an interrogation, which will help you achieve a better rapport with them. Finally, note how the answer concludes by broadening the subject onto other hobbies (no harm in reminding them!) and how they help you relieve pressure and stress.

Another example of an effective answer

One of the films that I particularly enjoyed watching was *Tea with Mussolini*, with Judy Dench, Maggie Smith and Cher. The film dealt with life in Italy during Mussolini's reign and particularly about the escape of an American Jewish woman played by Cher. It was a pleasant mix of historic reality and of comedy, which made it appealing to all ages. One of the things that I enjoyed about the film was the portrayal of solidarity between human beings in very difficult situations and the fact that those who had nothing to gain from the situation went out of their way to save the American Jewish woman. I also enjoyed the frequent references to art, through Judy Dench who was playing a mad artist based in Tuscany.

As well as watching films that have a historic base, I also enjoy comedies, adventure films and romantic films. Another film that I have enjoyed is *The English Patient*, which deals with the handling of human emotions. I enjoy going to the cinema with friends as well as watching videos. As well as helping me relieve stress, it gives me a good opportunity to socialise with my friends and colleagues.

9.38 This course requires a great deal of independent study. Will you manage?

In order to demonstrate that you can study independently, the best thing that you can do is to not speak hypothetically but to bring forward all your experience and your ability to organise yourself, plan your work and use all resources available to help you achieve your goals.

Be careful though; by talking about your independence, there is a small danger that you end up sounding selfish and like a loner. Although you want to demonstrate that you can study independently at university, you still have to show that you are flexible. The education system in Medicine is evolving all the time; it is important to have a flexible attitude towards your own education.

Example of an effective answer

For my GCSEs and in my sixth form, I was very independent in the way that I organised my studies. Obviously, I attended all lessons to gain a good understanding of each topic and I did all the homework required. I also took the initiative to gain information from different books about the topics that we were studying and by visiting related websites to broaden my understanding. Being able to study the same issues in different ways was very useful in giving me a thorough understanding of the topics.

I am a goal-oriented, organised and enthusiastic person and I study well on my own. I also find it interesting and relaxing to study in small groups. On occasions, when a topic was more difficult, I organised discussions with my friends so that we could think about the issue together.

Having already built up the culture of independent study, I feel that I can take this with me to my university education and be equally successful.

9.39 Studying for Medicine is a long and stressful process. What makes you think that you can cope with it?

This question is really about motivation and handling stress. The answer to it will therefore combine a number of elements that we have encountered in previous questions. Amongst other things, you will need to talk about:

- Your motivation for Medicine and your hard-working nature
- Your ability to handle stress and work well under pressure
- Your organisation skills and ability to multitask
- Your ability to seek help when necessary
- Your ability to work in teams and your sociability
- Your work-life balance.

You will need to raise each point in turn and back them up with personal examples that show that you have demonstrated those attributes.

Example of an effective answer

Going into Medicine is a decision that I have reached by myself having weighed the positives and negatives of the profession and I would not go into it if I did not feel that I could cope. I have always worked very hard in everything that I have done and working in an environment that is stressful and demanding is more likely to motivate me further than put me off Medicine. I have good organisation and time management skills, which helps me manage several tasks at the same time and ensures that I can plan my work ahead. For example, last year I was able to sail through my studies and achieve good marks and to find the time to have a Saturday job as well as my work experience and a couple of hobbies.

I get on well with people at all levels and, in particular, I find it easy to ask for assistance and advice when I need it. This means that, if I have a problem, I can find a way out very quickly, which saves time and worry. Finally, I have good mechanisms to deal with stress and pressure. I have learnt some very good relaxation techniques, which helped me through my A Levels. I also like playing music and doing drama, and I am hoping to be able to continue some of these activities at medical school. I am very close to my family and to a couple of very good friends and I know that they will provide me with the moral support that I will need during the next 5 years.

9.40 How would you make a patient feel less scared?

Why do patients get scared?

Before you can answer the actual question, you will need to discuss what may scare patients. This could be for example:

- The fear of dying
- The fear of needles
- The fear of stigma
- The fear of the unknown (i.e. they may never have been into hospital before and don't know how they will be treated)
- The fear of the impact a condition may have on their life (e.g. a professional driver diagnosed with epilepsy may not be able to drive again, thereby compromising his ability to make a living; this in turn may have other consequences (e.g. on marriage, mortgage, etc.))
- Mistrust in doctors or Medicine generally (e.g. following media stories)
- They are not thinking straight (e.g. they are confused, under the influence of medication, etc.)

If you can, try to give examples from your own experience as a patient or a relative, and from your work experience.

How do you deal with it?

In essence, the key to reassuring the patient will rest with your communication skills:

- Ensure that you ask the patient what they are scared about and why they are scared.

- Be an attentive listener and demonstrate empathy (this can be done by acknowledging their statements verbally: "I understand", "I can see you are feeling very strongly about this"; and through your body language: open body language, facing the patient, good eye contact, nodding in the right places).

- If necessary, explain to the patient the process again (e.g. the procedure or the course of treatment), making sure that they understand everything. Make sure you explain the issues in a language that the patient understands, with no or minimal jargon, using pictures/diagrams if necessary.

- If the patient remains scared, you might consider involving other people, for example an experienced nurse or a more senior doctor – some patients feel better when the words come from a consultant rather than a trainee.

- In some cases, it may also be appropriate to involve the relatives (making sure that the patient agrees so that there is no breach of confidentiality). For example, a woman about to give birth may be scared that something will happen to the baby. The presence and reassurance of the husband or a friend may help calm the patient down.

Again, if you can give an example of a situation where you have observed doctors dealing with a worried/scared patient or dealt with one yourself then you should do so.

9.41	One of your fellow students regularly misses lectures and tutorials, and stays in their room most of the time. What would you be concerned about? What would you do?

This question tests your ability to look at a situation from someone else's perspective and demonstrate empathy.

There are many reasons why a fellow student may behave in that way, such as:

- They are genuinely ill
- They are feeling isolated
- They are finding it hard to cope with the pressure of medical school
- They are lagging behind and turning up for lectures or tutorials may highlight their difficulties
- They have fallen out with someone they don't want to face
- They are depressed because of an external event (e.g. illness of a relative).

You may be concerned that:

- They are trying to deal with difficult issues on their own and do not have anyone to share their problems with
- They fall further behind in their studies
- They give up on studying Medicine
- They become depressed
- They overmedicate
- They commit suicide.

As a response you might consider:

- Visiting the student to make sure they are all right
- Asking if they need any assistance and if they need to talk
- Offering to help them catch up with the missed tutorials and lectures.

If you are very concerned:

- Discuss your concerns with someone responsible within the medical school (e.g. their educational supervisor or any tutor)
- Suggest that they seek professional help (e.g. see their GP or a counsellor – perhaps there are some at the medical school).

9.42 What are the reasons for people wanting cosmetic surgery?

When you are facing questions which relate to personal reasons and feelings, make sure you address them from the human perspective. In this particular case, answering "Some people want cosmetic surgery because their nose is too big or their breasts are too small" would be misplaced. What matters more is that you are able to see behind the obvious and demonstrate that you have a fundamental understanding of what drives people to make the choices they make.

In all such questions, it is important to consider three factors: physical, social and psychological.

Reasons why people may want cosmetic surgery include the following:

- They may be embarrassed by a particular feature (e.g. a deformity, large moles on their face, scars), and may even be the subject of bullying as a consequence. In some cases, this may make socialising difficult.

- They may be physically inconvenienced by a physical feature (e.g. laser surgery would mean no longer having to wear glasses, a breast reduction may reduce backache, removing a mole on the upper cheek will stop glasses rubbing on it).

- They have low self-esteem because they feel that some of their body parts are not aligned with their own expectations or their partner's expectations. Their expectations may have been distorted by the media.

- They are being pressured by someone else to undergo surgery (e.g. a partner asking for a specific procedure to be carried out).

- They are scared of getting/looking old. This may be fuelled by a fear of dying, a fear of losing their partner or a fear of not finding one.

- They are depressed and feel the need to "do something", a bit like shopping therapy.

- They are easily influenced and just want to follow a trend (e.g. having breast implants because all their friends have them).

9.43	A friend has asked your advice about how to tell her parents that she intends to drop out of university and go off travelling. How do you respond?

In your answer the interviewers will expect you to demonstrate that:

- You have empathy and a willingness to help your friend.
- You can advise her without being judgemental, without imposing your views and without being pushy.
- You can help your friend to come to her own conclusions.
- You attempt to understand the reasons which underlie the decision as opposed to simply judge the validity of her decision.
- You have an understanding of the parents' perspective.

Example of an effective answer

Rather than giving my own opinion straight off, I would like to explore with my friend why she feels she needs to make such a decision. It may be, for example, that she feels unsuccessful and stressed, or that she has been easily influenced by other factors. Having an open discussion about the motives behind her decision will help her crystallise her thoughts. That will then lead either to a change of mind or greater clarity about her decision. Throughout that discussion I would need to be careful not to pass judgement on her decisions.

One thing that would be of particular concern would be to make sure she has thought carefully of the consequences both on her own career and on how her parents feel. I would probably best address that by asking her open questions, and perhaps playing devil's advocate.

In terms of advising her on how to tell her parents, I would want to ask her what she anticipates their reactions to be as this may dictate the approach that will be required. For example, do you tell one parent first and then the other, or do you sit them both down at the same time? She will also need to make sure that there is time for discussion and that she is not simply dumping the news onto them without the means or time to debate the issue.

At the end of the day, the final decision as to how to approach her parents will be hers but the best I can do is to offer my support and ensure she approaches the issue with a cool head.

9.44   What makes you angry?

Fundamentally, though it would be perfectly normal to get angry about certain things, it never comes across well at an interview when you feel more nervous than usual. Stating issues that make you angry also risks landing you in a ping pong match with the interviewers of the type:

You: I get angry when people don't do what they are supposed to do.

Interviewer: That happens every day in Medicine. You will be permanently stressed if that makes you angry.

Or

You: The fact that there are millions of people on Earth without food and medicine makes me angry.

Interviewer: Given that you can't do much about it and that I can't see anything in your personal statement which indicates that you are trying to solve the problem, what is the point of getting angry about it?

Basically, you can't win, mainly because the word "angry" implies that you are fuming, being aggressive, shouting at people or, on the contrary, that you are bottling it up.

With this question, there are three important points to bear in mind:

1. It is safer to talk about things that "annoy" you rather than things that make you "angry". The point is to make the problem a frustration rather than something that deeply affects you psychologically.

2. You should only mention issues that you can learn to live with or that you can influence.

3. You should give examples of how you try to overcome your frustrations.

What can you talk about?

As long as you can put a positive spin on it and can show yourself in a good light, anything goes. It does help if you choose something realistic, particularly when it comes to giving an example.

Things that annoy you might include:

- Being delegated tasks by someone who is running behind schedule and is dumping their work onto you.

- People who go off on tangents in discussions.

- People who over-argue their points (i.e. don't move on, even when everyone agrees with them).

- Clock watchers.

- People who see problems in everything and never contribute any solutions.

- People who are judgemental.

- People who only care about themselves to the detriment of others.

- People who take credit for something someone else achieved.

- People who dismiss ideas without having even considered them.

- People who manipulate the truth to cover their own mistakes.

- Time wasting in meetings, with no structure or outcome to the discussions.

- Duplication of effort due to lack of communication.

Example of an effective answer

I can't say many things really make me angry. I tend to be fairly level-headed. But, like everyone else, there are things that can frustrate me greatly. One of those things is when you end up having to attend numerous meetings that go round in circles simply because people end up treating them as social occasions and tend to forget that the meeting was meant to be used to discuss specific issues with the aim to make a decision.

For example, I am interested in local politics and last year attended a meeting at my local council, where they were discussing issues to do with a planning application in relation to a car wash which had set up illegally down our road. The meeting went on for hours and it was clear that there was no real structure to it; as a result it became a free for all. At the end of the allocated 2 hours, no one was sure about what would happen next and the chairman simply mentioned that another meeting would be required to continue the discussions.

In normal circumstances (i.e. in circumstances where I am able to influence the situation – for example in a meeting with fellow students) I would try my best to ensure that the team stays focused on the discussions that were meant to happen, but in this instance it was not my place to interrupt. So I have found that the best thing to do when you can't control things is to be conscious that you can't actually change things but that the only thing you can control is your own frustration. So I try my best not to let it get to me.

10 Questions testing critical thinking (includes ethics)

10.1 In what ways can doctors promote good health other than through the direct treatment of an illness?

Doctors can promote good health by:

- Setting a good example to patients, for example by eating healthily, keeping fit and not smoking.

- During consultations, encouraging patients to have a healthy lifestyle (safe sex, no smoking, low fat diet, exercising, etc.).

- Displaying posters in their surgery and distributing leaflets to patients.

- Promoting support groups (smoking cessation, Alcoholics Anonymous).

- Recommending the services of a dietician.

However, health promotion goes well beyond this and also includes disease prevention and preventing the worsening of any existing illness a patient may have ("secondary prevention"). This includes:

- Screening programmes for target populations (e.g. breast cancers, cervical cancers, etc.).

- Immunisation campaigns and services.

- Family planning/sexual health clinics, well-women's/men's clinics and other specialist clinics (diabetes, etc.).

10.2 How does politics influence healthcare decisions?

There is an ongoing debate about whether the NHS would be better run by clinicians or by politicians. An argument in favour of clinicians is that they know best what patients need and the impact that decisions could have on the ground. An argument in favour of politicians is that the NHS is a public institution funded by taxpayers and that it is therefore only right that policy should be directed by people who have been elected by those who fund it.

Currently, politics has a major impact on the delivery of healthcare. Examples would include:

1. **Working hours:** the European Working Time Directive has substantially reduced the number of hours that a doctor can work (by limiting the working time of anyone who is employed to 48 hours per week). This has led to a need for more doctors, a need for better and more focused training and a need for a change in the role of other workers such as nurses, as well as a reorganisation of shift patterns. Further reforms may need to be implemented if European legislation imposes a degree of uniformity across all health systems around the EU.

2. **Funding:** the level of care that the NHS can provide is dictated by the budget that the government makes available. That budget comes from National Insurance contributions, which must be limited if the elected politicians do not want to incur the wrath of the electorate. Thus, for a politician, it is a trade-off between well-funded quality healthcare and not losing votes because of high taxes.

3. **Rationing:** because budgets are never enough to provide the full care that patients would expect, choices have to be made about how scarce resources should be allocated. Restrictions can be implemented in many ways; for example, by not allowing some categories of people to have access to certain drugs or surgery, or by not allowing some drugs or treatments on the NHS at all (e.g. most drugs used for cosmetic purposes). These are political decisions.

4. **Public health:** major awareness campaigns for issues of public importance can help the NHS pass on messages to the general public (e.g. the fight against sexually transmitted diseases, MMR vaccina-

tion, etc.) and can change public perception and behaviours. The allocation of budgets to different issues of interest may be dictated by the politics of the current government and personal beliefs of politicians.

5. **Regulation:** politics can also intervene indirectly; for example through the regulation of the pharmaceutical industry, which is a major source of funds for clinical research. There is a fine line between making sure that drugs are purchased at a reasonable price from companies so that best possible use can be made of taxpayers' money, while ensuring that pharmaceuticals retain the means to fund appropriate research.

10.3	Do you think it is right to allow private healthcare to run alongside the NHS?

You should ensure that you set out the pros and cons of private health-care before you give your own opinion. At the interview, make sure that you do not engage in political lobbying against the unfairness of a private sector reserved for the rich of this world. It may be unfair but there are two sides to the coin and you must demonstrate that you can show depth of thought, an open mind and the ability to present convincing arguments in a clear manner.

Arguments in favour of private healthcare

1. Private healthcare takes patients away from the NHS waiting lists. This means that NHS users can actually be treated more quickly as a result.

2. Those who use private healthcare facilities actually pay twice. They pay their standard National Insurance contributions and also have to pay for their healthcare privately on top of that. For the NHS, it means that the money can be redirected to other patients instead. Incidentally, at the last general election, the Conservatives were proposing that patients who used private healthcare should have part of their care paid for by the NHS. The idea was that they should benefit from part of the saving that the NHS made on them. The idea did not catch on at the time.

3. Some private healthcare is actually subcontracted back to the NHS (for example a private hospital may not be able to afford an MRI scanner and might send its patients to have it done at the local NHS hospital in exchange for payment). Similarly, some hospitals have private wards, which are rented to their doctors in the context of their private work.

4. Some doctors with higher ambitions want to supplement their income through private work. An impossibility to do private work could lead to doctors leaving Medicine, or leaving the country, or even taking on other jobs. All this would reduce their availability to the NHS (so-called "brain-drain").

5. The NHS cannot cope with all the demands placed upon it because of budgetary constraints. Introducing a private sector into the equation creates a market economy, which should drive efficiency and ultimately create better results. (Note that the trend is now to create a market economy within the health system, precisely for this reason – in particular, GPs will be able to refer patients to the NHS and the private sector alike, within set constraints.)

6. If there were no private healthcare sector in the UK, many people might go abroad to receive treatment. Any subsequent complications of substandard treatment would still have to be followed up by the NHS when patients return to the UK. One could therefore argue that you might as well treat patients where you can control the standard of care rather than having to deal with the consequences of their treatment abroad. If too many people went abroad, they might also refuse to pay their National Insurance contributions, which would have serious consequences for society and the NHS.

7. There is a fundamental issue of personal liberty and individual choice. Should a rich person be denied access to important care simply on the basis that a poorer person could not afford it and on the basis of equity?

Arguments against private healthcare

1. Private healthcare primarily benefits the wealthier part of the population or people who are employed by some of the bigger companies. This leads to inequality by selecting against the poorest (who also tend to be the neediest) – "The haves and the have-nots."

2. Some private institutions subcontract services back to the NHS. For example, a private hospital might send its patients to the local NHS hospital for an MRI scan, with those patients effectively buying priority slots and jumping queues. Also, there are so-called "private wards" in NHS hospitals, reserved for private patients of the NHS doctors working at that hospital. NHS doctors and nurses may still be called to these patients, e.g. in an emergency, which would take them away from their work. This inevitably diverts NHS time and resources away.

3. Because private healthcare is financially driven, there is an issue with the motivation of the doctor, which may not necessarily be altruistic. Also, with a financial incentive, doctors may be more inclined to follow

the patient's wishes rather than their best clinical judgement (i.e. have a commercial relationship). This motivation may also mean that patients are booked for investigations that may not be required (in a bid to extract money from insurance companies). Such investigations may even be detrimental to health (e.g. too much exposure to X-rays).

4. Time spent by doctors treating private patients would be better spent treating NHS patients. (In practice, this argument is a bit weak as such doctors would do their private work in their own time.)

5. Private healthcare does not provide full coverage. If a patient is in a private setting and requires intensive care urgently, this patient may be worse off as he may need to be transported to a better equipped establishment such as a local NHS hospital. The patient may suffer from this delay in implementing more dependent care.

Discussion

Once you have set out a range of pros and cons, you need to give your own opinion. This should be fairly balanced (some people on the panel may have a private practice while some others may be firmly against it). In fact, you may want to conclude that the arguments on both sides are so powerful that it is difficult to see how a definite answer could be given without upsetting half of the population.

10.4 How should healthcare be funded?

First of all, you must get out of your mind the fact that there is a right or a wrong answer to this. This question is an ongoing question in politics and, if they have been fighting over it for dozens of years in Parliament, you won't find the answer in 2 minutes at an interview.

What this question is really asking you is whether you can have a small debate between the various options, which takes us back primarily to the previous question: "Do you think it is right to allow private healthcare to run alongside the NHS?" However, it may be an idea to have some basic knowledge of what is going on around the world too. Here are a few broad examples:

Scandinavia: healthcare is funded solely by taxpayers. As a result, taxation is high and private healthcare is not very prominent.

USA: the majority of healthcare provision is through the private sector and only the poor are treated by the State. Everyone else must have insurance cover to fund their own healthcare.

France: Mixed system. Taxation is high to finance a public system used by everyone. Individual practitioners charge whatever they wish for each consultation or treatment. A set tariff is reimbursed to the patient by the State. The difference between the actual fee and the reimbursed tariff is picked up by a private insurance company if the patient has taken out excess insurance.

Ultimately, every system has its advantages and its flaws. Every system is constantly criticised either for being too expensive, too unfair, too inefficient or too open to abuse. In addition, local culture plays an important part in deciding what different societies find acceptable. For example, a US-style system would be difficult to introduce in Europe where social protection is high on the agenda.

10.5 What do you think of the way doctors are perceived in the media?

There is a tendency for candidates to view the media's perception of doctors as negative. In a sense, a degree of negativity is inevitable since happy events do not make exciting news unless they are truly outstanding, while the slightest negative anecdote can make front page news. The ongoing occurrence of various scandals (Shipman, Northwick Park research trials, Mid-Staffordshire NHS Trust, etc.) does not help their cause either.

You must first present the different points of view before discussing your opinion. And don't forget that the term "media" includes a wide range of media and not just tabloid newspapers.

Positive portrayal of doctors in the media

- Heroic events such as the role of doctors and paramedics during the aftermath of the 7 July 2005 bombings.
- Pioneering operations such as the separation of conjoined twins.
- Important discoveries such as a possible vaccine for cervical cancer. (Although such discoveries are not always made by doctors, but often by research scientists, they are often associated with clinicians in the public's mind.)
- Glorifying and glamorising doctors through well-known TV series, showing amazing feats of deduction, clinical skills and procedures in a dramatised fashion, presenting doctors as god-like characters.
- Fly-on-the-wall documentaries that show real-life doctors doing day-to-day caring, where the viewers can easily relate to the patients.

Negative portrayal of doctors in the media

- Dr Shipman killing numerous patients (see Section 5.1).
- Major scandals such The Bristol Heart Hospital Scandal, organ retention scandal at Alder Hey Hospital (Liverpool), clinical research going wrong at Northwick Park Hospital, failure of the Trust at Mid-Staffordshire, etc.
- Controversial topics such as MMR and autism (see Section 5.2).
- Doctors involved in botched operations and generally any GMC investigation related in the media.
- Financial gains made by doctors (private practice, GP salaries).

- Going on strike to defend own pension rights when public perception is that doctors are highly paid.

What do you think about the portrayal of doctors?

In your discussion about the portrayal of doctors, you will need to discuss whether the portrayal is correct and fair. Arguments that you may wish to develop include:

- The media is using information to generate sales or advertising. Therefore the tendency is to present newsworthy items, which are often at the two extremes of the spectrum (either very positive or very negative). This may give people the wrong impression about doctors. Very positive news may raise expectations beyond reason. Very negative news may decrease public confidence.

- The media plays an important role in highlighting the flaws of the system and exposing faulty practices. This ensures that the system does not cover up any wrongdoing and that doctors stick to a behaviour characterised by personal integrity.

- The media plays an important role in debating important health issues and in questioning political decisions. For example, the controversy about the MMR vaccine was fuelled by the media in search of the truth. This forced all parties to reveal their evidence, and increased transparency. This quest for transparency keeps doctors alert, and ensures that they remain accurate in the messages that they convey to the public.

10.6 What does the phrase "inequalities in healthcare" mean to you?

Inequalities in healthcare occur when individuals or groups are not treated in the same manner as others in similar situations. There are several ways in which inequalities in healthcare manifest themselves, which we have set out below. In your answer, you should address a handful of these points (and others that you may have derived for yourself). Do not just list them, but expand on them a little to show an understanding of the issues.

Socio-economic inequalities

Parts of the population are less educated than others and consequently have a poorer understanding of their own health needs and poor awareness of the availability of appropriate services. This has several consequences:

- Common health prevention messages may not find their way to the individuals concerned (avoiding unwanted pregnancies, smoking cessation, healthy eating, living and lifestyle). For this reason, the government is enhancing health promotion targeting through the appropriate media.

- Available services may not be used to their optimum by people in such vulnerable groups. The government is promoting a drive to increase the level of services being provided in a community setting, which should address part of that problem.

Similar arguments and solutions exist for other minority groups based on ethnicity, language barriers and immigration status.

Geographical distribution of healthcare resources

This is commonly referred to as the "postcode lottery". It refers to the fact that individuals are receiving different levels of care depending on the region in which they live. For example:

- There is a geographic concentration of resources and skills. People living in urban areas have easier access to healthcare facilities (including GPs) than people living in cities.

245

- Primary Care Trusts can make independent decisions about the provision of treatment based on their available budgets. This can mean that treatments available in one Trust may not be made available in another Trust.

Public healthcare vs. private healthcare

See Q.10.3 for comprehensive arguments.

10.7 What are the arguments for and against people paying for their own healthcare?

Be careful with this question. Its wording suggests that it is not about public vs. private sectors (see Q.10.3) but about what the consequences would be of moving from the current insurance-based system in the UK to a system whereby patients would pay for their healthcare as and when they need it (as if they were going shopping). If in doubt, ask the interviewers to clarify what they mean.

Arguments for paying for your own healthcare

1. Currently, you pay National Insurance contributions whether you need the NHS or not. Under this other system you would only pay for what you need. This would be a distinct advantage if your health is good.

2. It would prevent time-wasting patient visits (e.g. patients going to the GP for a simple cold) as patients would only go if they really needed to.

3. It would introduce competition at doctors' level, which would lead to a "fight" for your custom and therefore increased standards of care.

4. It may encourage people to have healthier lifestyles in order to minimise the need to use healthcare facilities.

Arguments against paying for your own healthcare

1. It would place the poorest at a clear disadvantage. Not only are they the neediest group, they are also those who could afford healthcare the least.

2. Knowing that they have to pay, some patients may put off going to see a doctor or may not go at all. This may cause problems if medical attention is urgently required.

3. This may encourage situations whereby doctors refuse to treat patients until payment has been made, even in cases of emergency (there have been cases in the US where doctors refused to admit patients until someone could produce a credit card).

4. With a choice between several possible treatments or procedures, patients may choose the cheapest available as opposed to one with the best outcome.

5. Patients with chronic illnesses would face spiralling costs, at a time when they may also be out of work.

6. It would create a relationship between the doctor and the patient that is based on money. This may affect the doctor's integrity as he may be more inclined to follow the patient's wishes rather than what he feels is best for the patient.

7. Unscrupulous doctors could take advantage of the process by organising more investigations than required or referring patients to their friends.

8. Some patients may turn to cheaper alternatives such as some forms of alternative medicines, which may not be adequate or even safe for their condition.

9. It may encourage a black market in health practices, which would be unregulated and dangerous for patients (see, for example, the practice of backstreet abortions before abortion was legalised).

10.8   What are alternative medicines/complementary therapies? What is your opinion of them?

What are alternative medicines/complementary therapies?

These terms apply to therapies that are different to conventional medicine, i.e. the Medicine taught at medical schools in the UK. They tend to be given by non-medical practitioners, although some doctors now integrate some of these therapies within their practice. They can come in many forms, including:

- Homeopathy
- Acupuncture
- Aromatherapy
- Reflexology

- Hypnosis
- Herbalism
- Chinese Medicine
- Crystals

The terms "alternative" and "complementary" apply to all these types of therapy but are distinguished by the way in which they are used.

Alternative Medicine = therapy taken <u>instead of</u> conventional treatment.
Complementary therapy = therapy taken <u>alongside</u> conventional treatment.

At an interview, you would be wise to make it clear that you understand the distinction and address both of these contexts despite what the question might be, as those terms are often wrongly used interchangeably.

Arguments for

1. Some therapies involve a high level of contact between the therapist and the patient. The time spent treating the patient is often considerably longer than a conventional doctor's consultation and may have a beneficial effect on the patient.

2. Many therapies do not involve taking substances into the system and therefore there is a low level of side effects experienced by the patient.

3. Some therapies involve a spiritual component which, along with the greater therapist-patient relationship, may fulfil the needs of patients who require a more holistic approach to their care.

4. When conventional medicine is failing a patient or where options have run out, alternative therapies can offer further hope.

5. Although they may not necessarily treat the underlying medical condition, they may still have a role in treating side effects of conventional treatments or complications of the underlying condition.

Arguments against

1. The evidence base backing these therapies is not as substantial as compared to the evidence available for conventional medicine. The evidence is mostly based on anecdotes or small controlled series, not all of which have been shown to be reproducible. This is weak compared to the stringent standards imposed on research for conventional medicine.

2. Conventional medicine rests on scientific principles of pathophysiology whereas the mechanism of action of alternative therapies is often poorly understood.

3. Some complementary therapies involve taking substances that may be toxic (such as liver toxicity of some Chinese Medicine treatments) or that may interact with conventional treatments being taken simultaneously.

4. Currently, alternative therapies are poorly regulated, if at all. This has allowed charlatans to abuse the trust of some of their patients.

5. In most cases, an alternative therapist will not be a trained conventional doctor and, therefore, will not be in a position to advise the patient with the full picture in mind. This may lead to patients making ill-informed and sometimes harmful decisions.

10.9 Do you think the NHS should provide alternative therapies?

Alternative therapies are a sensitive topic and doctors can have very extreme views on this matter. Those views are often linked to personal pride, personal experience and anecdotes, or ignorance of the facts.

At an interview, you will not be judged on your personal views but on the manner in which you bring together your arguments to reach a conclusion. All in all, it helps to keep an open mind, particularly when there are so many unknowns about the topic and when some doctors are starting to practise alternative therapy alongside their conventional practice.

How to answer the question
If you say yes, they will throw at you all the negative aspects of alternative medicine identified in the answer to Q.10.8. If you say no, they will do the same with the positive aspects.

The only sensible answer to this question is: "It depends on whether the NHS can get around all the negative aspects." You should therefore list those negative aspects (see Q.10.8) and explain what would be needed to get around these. This would include:

- More research (i.e. widening the evidence base)
- Better knowledge of mechanism (also widening the evidence base)
- Understanding of harmful effects and compatibility with current treatments
- Improved regulation
- Adequate training
- Ensuring that alternative practitioners also have a conventional medical background.

10.10   Should the NHS deal with patients who have self-inflicted diseases?

Many candidates have a narrow understanding of this question and spend 2 minutes talking about suicide and other forms of self-harm. These are not self-inflicted <u>diseases</u>.

Another misinterpretation is to discuss how the NHS currently deals with self-inflicted diseases. This question is not about what the current status is. It is asking for a debate about whether it should deal with such patients.

What are self-inflicted diseases?

Some common conditions include:
- Skin cancer following prolonged exposure to sun-rays
- Obesity following bad dietary habits
- Lung cancer due to smoking
- Liver cirrhosis following excessive drinking
- HIV following conscious high risk-taking behaviour
- Hepatitis C following injected drug use
- Heart disease and hypertension following an unhealthy lifestyle.

In favour of the NHS dealing with self-inflicted diseases

1. The large majority of diseases are self-inflicted to some extent, even though the link may not be obvious. Indeed, bar a small number of genetically inherited diseases, most are linked in one way or another to our lifestyle. Excluding self-inflicted conditions would restrict a health system to treating only a minority of conditions.

2. It follows from the above that most of us will need to see a doctor for an issue that will bear some relation to our lifestyle. Public perception would be greatly damaged if we could not get help for some of the most common diseases.

3. Assuming that we may want to exclude some self-inflicted diseases from NHS care, it would be difficult to determine the extent to which a disease is self-inflicted and therefore whether it should be treated or not. (Consider, for example, the case of a woman who had unpro-tected sex with her long-term husband because she trusted him, but where the husband acquired HIV through a one-night stand and re-

fused to notify his wife. Would you say that the wife's HIV was self-inflicted? How would you know that she is not lying simply to get treatment?)

4. On public health grounds, it is necessary to treat any transmissible diseases (such as sexually transmitted diseases), to control them and to prevent onward transmission.

5. Some self-inflicted behaviours (such as excessive drinking or smoking) may reveal underlying issues (e.g. psychiatric conditions or psychological ill-being) that may need to be identified and treated. Not allowing patients to visit a doctor for a self-inflicted illness may prevent the treatment of those underlying causes.

6. We are in a free society where individual choice is of crucial importance. The NHS should complement this society choice and not work against it.

Against

1. Patients with self-inflicted diseases often relapse. They may feel that they have got away with it before and return to their high risk behaviours. Treating them might therefore be only a temporary measure for a problem which may recur later on, e.g. ongoing sexually risky behaviour, alcoholism relapse following liver transplant.

2. Allowing treatment of self-inflicted diseases may remove individual responsibility for one's own health. For example, people will not consider some behaviour as high risk in the first place because they know that they will receive treatment if they need to. In some cases (such as drug-related conditions), treating patients may actually be seen as encouraging illegal activities.

3. In a system where resources are scarce, it is important to prioritise how budgets need to be allocated. Public perception of the health service may be worsened if they see people who are less deserving in their eyes receive treatment when they themselves are struggling to be treated. This is an argument that the media used a lot in relation to the use of lottery funds. Much fuss was made about the fact that some funds were allocated to charities dealing with transsexuals and refugees, amongst others.

Important conclusion to raise

Ultimately, it is down to society to decide how it wants to use its own health system and, in particular, if it wishes to refuse treatment to individuals whose diseases are or appear to be self-inflicted.

Based on the arguments above, it would be very difficult to separate with certainty self-inflicted from non-self-inflicted diseases and therefore such an exclusion system would not be fair or practical.

10.11 Should alcoholics and smokers receive equal treatment to those who don't drink and don't smoke?

This question deals primarily with the issue of self-inflicted diseases. The arguments for this are contained in our answer to Q.10.10.

The question of whether alcoholics and smokers should be treated equally also brings into play the scarcity of resources available to the health system. In an ideal world where resources are abundant, the question would simply not arise as there would be enough to deal with everyone. In fact, it could even be argued that alcoholics and smokers need more help than others in many respects. In particular, it is worth recognising that addiction is a psychological/psychiatric condition in itself, which would benefit from extra help from the health system and from you as a doctor.

10.12 What are the arguments for and against the sale of tobacco?

Arguments for:

1. People should have the right to choose what is good for them. It is their choice to take a health risk.

2. Tobacco sales generate revenue through heavy taxation. This revenue can be used for the benefit of society as a whole.

3. Banning the sale of tobacco would lead to the development of a black market and would make the consequences uncontrollable. People with tobacco-linked illness would not dare seek medical assistance for fear of being prosecuted, which could have an overall negative effect on society.

4. Tobacco farmers (often in poor countries) rely heavily on those sales to survive. Banning tobacco would have a devastating effect on parts of the world economy.

5. Some people argue that tobacco is a drug, but then so is alcohol or hamburgers to some people (with equally devastating effects). So why not allow the sale of tobacco?

Arguments against:

1. Tobacco leads to serious respiratory diseases. This drains NHS resources and effectively wipes out the benefit of the additional revenue gained through taxation.

2. Not only is the smoker exposed, other people are exposed to secondary smoking. They do not have the same choice that smokers have. This includes babies, who may develop an addiction themselves through passive exposure and start smoking later on in life.

3. Addiction to cigarettes might lead to addiction to stronger drugs later.

4. Cigarette ends sometimes litter the streets, creating an unhygienic and dirty environment (see some famous capitals in Europe for reference).

Discussion

Ultimately, there is no denying that the sale of tobacco is crucial in bringing additional revenue into the economy, though heavy taxes also act as a regulator. A total ban would be impossible to impose without putting in place a police state; hence governments need to find a way to control the situation with a happy medium.

Smoking is a form of self-harm and to that extent it could be argued that it is the individual's responsibility to regulate his own consumption. Governments and other organisations are working hard at reconciling the various conflicting interests and actions are being taken on different counts:

- **Informed choice:** individuals may smoke at will but efforts are being made to ensure that they are aware of the consequences of smoking (campaigns on lung cancer, unsavoury messages on packets, etc.).

- **Prevention:** other than the dissemination of information about smoking, the government has tackled the issue of passive smoking by introducing a partial ban on smoking in places where food is being served. Several countries have introduced bans on smoking in public places.

10.13 How do you go about researching something you know nothing about?

There may be occasions where you will be asked to research an unknown topic, not least if you have the opportunity to get into a medical school that uses problem-based learning as a teaching tool, but also in your professional life where you may be asked to give presentations about topics that may be new to you and require a degree of homework.

Every candidate will have experience of dealing with topics with which they are unfamiliar and so it is best if you give examples of real-life situations to illustrate your points. Incidentally, your answer does not have to be constrained to the field of Medicine.

If you don't know something, the answer will either be in a book or journal, or in someone else's brain. To get answers you might therefore want to try the following:

- Talk to people who are experts in the field or have undertaken a similar type of research previously
- Look on the internet and in specialist medical databases
- Consult journals and magazines. Look in books.

Example of an effective answer

I was particularly interested in Herceptin recently; I kept hearing about it but knew nothing about the drug. I started off finding out about the medication from various daily newspapers. I also asked my GP and my biology teacher about the drug and the controversies surrounding it. This gave me the idea to go to the library, where I found out about monoclonal antibodies and how they are used to tackle breast cancer cell receptor HER2. I also used the internet to find out about the controversies surrounding the licensing of the drug and the various court cases that took place as a result. Using all these resources gave me a lot of information about the topic and talking with others allowed me to put everything in perspective. In the process I also learnt quite a lot about the process of drug licensing and breast cancer in general.

10.14 How do you know what you don't know?

Once you have recovered from the shock of the question's wording, you need to clarify in your mind what it means. Essentially, as a student, and later as a doctor, you will have gaps in your knowledge.

There will be things that you know are missing from your knowledge; in which case you will need to find ways of gaining that missing knowledge. There will also be things that you don't know and that you didn't even know existed. For these, you will need to do some digging to identify what you should have known in the first place.

Identifying gaps in your knowledge

There are many ways in which you identify gaps in your knowledge:

- Assessing yourself against a known list of criteria (syllabus, tick list of skills to acquire, common level of competence for peers).
- Obtaining feedback from others.
- Through experience. You see someone who does something that you can't do or knows something that you don't know but that you feel you should know.
- Taking account of complaints and comments.
- Learning from your mistakes and bad experiences.

Remedying your weaknesses

Once you have explained how you go about identifying what you don't know then you should explain the steps that you take to bridge the gap. This could include:

- Seeking advice and learning from colleagues.
- Attending suitable courses (in-house or external).
- Applying for suitable exams.
- Reading books or finding information on the internet.
- Observing others.
- Working extra time to gain more experience.
- Taking the initiative to get involved in activities or projects where you will gain further experience and confidence.

10.15 Should the NHS fund non-essential surgery?

The best approach for questions such as these is to see whether you can start answering by defining some of the key terms. When you look at the question, you should be asking yourself what "non-essential" means. By discussing this term, you will get ideas that you can develop during your answer.

What does non-essential mean?

Most people relate the concept of non-essential to cosmetic surgery. Although cosmetic surgery probably constitutes the bulk of it, there are other interventions that would qualify too. The concept of "non-essential" is ambiguous in itself as well as subjective. What may be regarded as non-essential by someone may be essential for someone else. For example, take a moment to think about the following cases:

- If a good-looking woman wants to have cosmetic surgery on her nose because she thinks that it is too big and is depressed as a result, does it constitute non-essential surgery? What if this would cure her depression?

- If a woman has breasts so large that she gets backache as a result, would breast reduction be essential surgery?

- What about a man with very thick glasses requiring laser surgery because he cannot stand the weight of his glasses any longer and his eyes are too dry to wear contact lenses?

- What about a 40-year-old man who requests a vasectomy because he already has four children and does not want to use condoms? What if he later wants a reversal of his vasectomy? Should this be funded by the NHS too?

Arguments in favour of funding non-essential surgery

1. Although some procedures may look like non-essential, the problem may affect the patients deeply from a psychological point of view. Carrying out a surgical procedure may prove more effective than letting the psychological problem progress further, with a potential risk of de-

veloping into a depression that may prove more expensive to resolve later.

2. Not funding non-essential surgery pushes people to self-fund the surgery, which may lead to significant debts for the patient.

3. Not funding may push people to choose to have surgery in other less regulated environments. This could have consequences on the NHS if patients then need help from the NHS to deal with complications.

Arguments against funding non-essential surgery

1. Requests for some non-essential treatments such as cosmetic surgery may only be the result of a deeper primary problem such as lack of self-esteem or depression, which may be treated better through psychological or psychiatric intervention. Treating the underlying problem may also be more suitable because cosmetic surgery is unlikely to resolve the psychological problem and the patient will slide down a slippery slope, requiring more and more surgery.

2. Knowing that treatment for non-essential surgery is available free of charge, people may find new problems to which they never paid attention before (e.g. a woman who had no problems with her breasts but now feels that she may as well have them enlarged).

3. Whereas non-essential surgery results from a request driven by the individual's own initiative, the need for essential surgery is driven by external events (e.g. a disease, an accident, etc.). As a result, the need for essential surgery can be reasonably anticipated from one year to the next, but allowing non-essential surgery to be funded by the NHS would open floodgates. This would lead to a gridlock situation and/or a need for additional funding. This in turn would lead to an increase in taxes, which would be shared by all taxpayers. Everyone would pay for other people's non-essential surgery, which would be unfair for those who do not require it.

10.16 Would you say that Medicine is an art or a science?

Before you can answer this question, it is crucial to have a good under-standing of what these two terms mean. There are many possible defini-tions for "science", but essentially it is the systematic acquisition of knowl-edge that is verifiable and a process for evaluating empirical knowledge. Art, on the other hand, is the product of creativity or imagination.

It would be too easy to think of Medicine as a science simply based on the fact that it is all about accumulating a vast number of facts about a topic based on observation and experimentation. The application of that knowl-edge is not as straightforward as it seems and, in many ways, makes Medicine closer to an art than a science. For example:

- Communicating with patients in order to gain a proper history can be a challenge. In many cases, there will be protocols to follow (which would make the process scientific) but patients do not always respond in accordance to theory. Extracting that information may require some ingenuity and creativity, making it an art.

- In general, anything to do with communication is an art as you need to adapt to the person or group that you are addressing. Breaking bad news to a patient is an art that not many doctors master, in the same way that being an effective teacher is an art. In particular, neither can be easily reproduced as patients and students are all different.

- Medicine also involves leading and managing teams that will help you provide the best care for your patients. Although there are manage-ment theories that you may apply, such a role relates more to a form of art where you have to use your imagination to resolve complex situations such as conflict or demotivated colleagues. The intervention of human feelings in the equation makes all the difference.

- There are some more obvious relationships between art and Medi-cine; for example a surgeon's ability to close a wound without leaving a scar, or the obvious sculpting skills of a plastic surgeon.

Nothing is ever as simple as it looks. It is fair to say that Medicine com-bines aspects of both art and science. Your answer should reflect this.

10.17 How do you solve the problem of transplant organ shortage?

There are only two approaches that you can take to solving the problem of transplant organ shortages:

1. Remove the need for transplants of living organs by increasing research to find alternative solutions to using real organs (e.g. grow organs on demand, use animal organs or find alternative cures for diseases).

2. Increase the number of organs being donated. This is probably the most realistic and quickest-to-implement option. The question is: how do you go about it?

Possible solutions to increase donations

For many reasons (religious, psychological, etc.), many people feel very uncomfortable donating organs to others, even if these organs are removed after their death. The problem is even more acute when it comes to donating organs while alive. Mostly, so far, the principle has been that organs could only be taken with the consent of the donor or the family in some cases. This relies heavily on people's altruism, which is in short supply, and on potential donors carrying cards on their person.

Other than encouraging people to carry donor cards, several other suggestions have been made and sometimes implemented around the world:

Imposing that everyone should be a donor

Although this would inevitably resolve the issue, it poses serious ethical dilemmas. Essentially, if patients can invoke their autonomy when they are alive, why should they not be allowed to decide what happens to them when they are dead? For some people, this also raises religious issues, which cannot be discounted.

Financial incentives

Paying for organs is currently illegal in the UK because it is open to abuse and would lead to the establishment of the traffic in organs, which could have devastating effects on parts of the population. Individuals would seek to obtain organs from poorer countries to sell them at a profit back in the UK; poorer individuals in the UK would also offer their organs for sale simply to make ends meet. The main problem is the direct payment of money against an organ, which could create a market with a totally different set of values (e.g. some people would profit from other people's misery). However, other less direct solutions were tried or proposed around the world, including:

- Giving discounts on driving licences for those who wish to become an organ donor ($9 discount in Georgia, USA).

- Establishing a market for options on organs. Under this principle, a potential donor would sell the right to his organs for a small amount of money. Once the donor dies, then his estate/family would receive a larger sum of money if the organs are actually used. The advantage of this solution is that the organ is not actually purchased from the donor immediately and the future donor only gets a small sum of money. Therefore it eliminates the risk of organ trafficking and the risk of poorer people selling body parts for immediate cash (since the amount will not be substantial enough in relation to the sacrifice). Another advantage is that it is the donor who actually makes the decision. Since it is the family that will benefit, it could almost be viewed as some kind of life insurance plan.

Reciprocity plans

These plans are already in place in the US (see www.lifesharers.com for an example) and are sometimes called no-give-no-take plans. Essentially, they are members' clubs which you join if you have organs that you want to donate. In exchange, you are entitled to receive organs from members of the club too. The system works on a point system to determine who is entitled to what benefit. In principle, such plans look like a good idea and get around the issue of financial incentive by encouraging altruism. However, they discriminate against people who are in poor health or who have no/few organs that may be fit for transplant.

Ultimately, the most realistic and immediate manner in which to increase donations will be to find ways of de-stigmatising death and encouraging people to get over the psychological barrier of donating organs to others. This is very much a communications exercise for the government and the NHS to undertake in order to change mentalities.

10.18 Ten years ago, most doctors wore white coats. Now, few of them do. Why is that?

There are two issues to consider for this question.

Infection control

Essentially, white coats were originally designed as clothes protectors and to minimise the risk of infections as they are easy to wash often (unlike suits that have to be dry-cleaned). It was also a good way for doctors to differentiate themselves (perhaps an ego trip, but also useful in emergencies).

Doctor-patient relationship

In an era where the patient is at the centre of the care, the relationship between patient and doctor has taken an increased importance and in many cases it was felt that the white coat created an artificial barrier to that relationship. In an effort to get closer to their patients and to appear more professional, many doctors have dropped the white coat in favour of the more traditional suit and tie (except some GPs who, in a further effort to get even closer to their patients, do not always bother with the tie).

Although wearing a suit has a definite advantage in terms of bringing doctors and patients closer, it also has a number of disadvantages.

- First of all, not all patients like to see their doctor in a suit. For many (particularly the elderly), the white coat symbolised a scientific authority and offered reassurance.

- Secondly, a suit is not easy to clean on a daily basis. With doctors wearing stethoscopes around their neck all day and with their tie brushing on various patients throughout the day, a suit poses an infection risk (hence recent debates about whether doctors should wear ties or not).

In fact, nowadays, for infection control reasons, many trusts have banned white coats, suits, ties (they rub on patients when you lean over), any garment with long-shirt sleeves and any jewellery at risk of coming into contact with patients.

10.19	Why do you think that life expectancy in the north of England is 5 years less than in the south according to statistics?

The danger with this question is to rush into a simplistic answer of the type: "That is because there are fewer healthcare facilities in the north." Although it may be true because there are more rural areas than in the south, surely it cannot account for such a big difference in life expectancy.

Here is one way of analysing the question:

Q: What are the biggest killers in the UK?
A: Lung cancer and heart disease.

Q: What are the main causes of lung cancer and heart disease?
A: Smoking and bad diet.

Q: Who is more likely to smoke and have an unhealthy diet?
A: People on lower incomes.

Q: Why would there be more people on lower incomes in the north?
A: Because it is more industrial and unemployment is higher than in the more affluent south.

Obviously, this approach is very general but it does help raise some important issues, which you can use to start building an answer.

As well as smoking and diet, there are other factors that may play a role, although most likely at a lower level. Here are some arguments that you can develop:

1. Statistics are often calculated over periods of several years. In particular, in order to measure the life expectancy at birth, you would need to wait until everyone from a particular year of birth has died. Therefore, the figure of 5 years is likely to include many people who were born a long time ago when living conditions were different. The 5 years quoted in the question may not be representative of the life expectancy of a baby who is being born now. For new-born babies, the difference in life expectancy taking account of changes in lifestyle over the years may well be lower than 5 years.

2. The north of England has traditionally been industrial and many in-
    habitants are on lower incomes than in the south. For many, this has
    led to a culture of excessive smoking and unhealthy diet, which itself
    has led to lung cancer and heart disease. This has undoubtedly been
    compounded by stress in many instances, due to having to raise fami-
    lies in difficult circumstances including threats of redundancy and un-
    employment. People in the south tend to be more affluent (more ser-
    vice-based industries) and tend to have healthier lifestyles both in
    terms of smoking and diet.

3. Lower income is also associated with lesser awareness of health is-
    sues. People in the north on average may therefore be less receptive
    to health messages than in the south. Lower awareness and under-
    standing of health issues may also mean a lower level of compliance
    with medication once it has been prescribed.

4. Climate may have an impact on psychological well-being. The highest
    rates of suicide in the world are in Lithuania, Russia, Belarus, Latvia,
    etc. There are strong suspicions that climate plays an important role.
    This may also affect people living in the north of England, with possi-
    bly more depression and suicidal tendencies (note: this is purely
    speculative!).

5. Access to healthcare may be greater in the south than in the north, as
    there are more rural areas in the north and services in the south are
    more concentrated.

6. People in the south are more affluent and therefore have better ac-
    cess to stress-relieving activities and luxuries including holidays, gym
    membership, etc.

Be very careful not to generalise too much though, as you might appear
bigoted. Bear in mind that we are just talking in terms of statistics here and
not individual by individual. We are not saying that everyone in the north
smokes, eats badly, is unemployed or on low income, and is uneducated.
We are talking about trends and averages covering parts of the population. If you compare individual to individual, you might even find that, for
example, a lawyer in the north has a higher life expectancy than in the
south because he will have a better quality of life.

10.20 Why do you think it is that we cannot give a guarantee that a medical treatment or surgical procedure will be successful?

What does successful mean?

First of all you would need to ask yourself how you define success for a surgical procedure or a medical treatment. For example, someone who needs a hip replacement may walk very well thereafter. But what if a degree of pain subsists or they limp slightly? Someone who undertakes a medical treatment may well have their original condition treated but what if the medication taken has given rise to severe side effects or, worse, to another condition? Success is not always a black-and-white concept.

In addition, you need to ask yourself whether success means success for the patient or for the doctor. A doctor will define success according to his experience and his original intentions for giving the treatment or undertaking the procedure. A patient may consider other parameters too, in accordance with their own expectation prior to treatment/procedure. For example:

- A patient may view success in relation to how much of their original lifestyle they have been able to recommence, or in relation to the degree of autonomy that they have.

- A laser eye operation that only corrects part of the patient's eyesight may be viewed as a medical success because the operation achieved a result well within the norm. But, to a patient who may have hoped for a total correction and an end to wearing spectacles, this may appear to be a failure.

- A surgical operation that leaves a visible scar may be viewed as a success because it achieved its original aim, but the patient may view the remaining scar as a sign of failure or at least a lesser success.

Patient-linked factors

The success of a surgical operation or a medical treatment depends on many patient-related factors. In particular:

1. The patient may not have revealed all the relevant information during the history-taking process, therefore leading doctors to make a deci-

sion on incomplete information. This would result in the proposed treatment not being entirely suitable.

2. The physical well-being of the patient at the time of the treatment or procedure is important. This could include physical characteristics or any pre-existing conditions which may interfere with the success of the treatment. For example, obesity may make a surgical procedure more complex, thereby rendering the process more risky; a smoker may have fragile skin, which enhances the risk of scarring after surgery.

3. On the medical side, the proposed treatment may not have the desired result on the patient. For example, this may be because the patient is simply not responding to the treatment, because the patient has built resistance over time or because the treatment interferes with another current treatment.

4. The patient may not adhere to the medical treatment or post-operative medication. This could be for many reasons, including the fear of side effects, the fear of a negative impact on lifestyle, the pain of having to count and take a large number of pills every day, etc.

5. The patient may develop complications that may have an adverse effect on the success of the treatment or the procedure.

Doctor-linked factors

1. The surgeon may not be fully competent in the procedure or in managing the condition, thus making it difficult for him to deal with adverse consequences. This could be through lack of training/exposure or because the case is rare.

2. The doctor may have made the wrong diagnosis.

3. Not all treatments work on all people (a simple example is that paracetamol clears some people's headaches and not other people's). Often doctors prescribe a first line of treatment and then, if that doesn't work, they increase the dose or switch the patient to a new treatment. The doctor would therefore not wish to guarantee success.

10.21 What do you think would be the advantages, and difficulties, for a person with a major physical disability (e.g. blindness) wishing to become a doctor?

Advantages

1. People whose disability has affected one of their senses severely often compensate by having another sense more developed. For example, a blind person may have developed better hearing and a stronger listening ability, which could help in a medical setting. Similarly, someone who is unable to walk may have developed a stronger dexterity, which could be useful in carrying out procedures and surgery.

2. Blind people have also often developed an ability to retain, analyse and process information efficiently. This could prove very useful during their studies and later on during their medical career.

Difficulties

1. Major disabilities could cause serious problems for day-to-day aspects of medical care. For example, someone who cannot walk would find it difficult to attend to a patient in an emergency. A blind person would not be able to examine a patient in depth and spot important clinical signs without help from other colleagues; they would also not be in a position to ensure that they are administering the correct drug at the right dosage to a patient.

2. A blind student would find it difficult to learn as fast as his colleagues as he would need to transcribe all his notes in a readable format.

Discussion

Ultimately, there is a place in Medicine for most people, even some of the more severely disabled. Although they will of course not be in a position to take on responsibilities where their disability would endanger patient safety, there are posts that offer real prospects, either because they can be carried out with the help of others (after all a blind person could perform well as a medic if he had a suitable assistant acting as his/her eyes) or because their work is of a more academic nature.

10.22 **Do charities have a role in society or do you think that the government should decide where all the money should go?**

Consequences of giving charities a role

1. Individuals exercise personal responsibility by contributing directly to the advancement of causes that matter to them. Individuals can direct funds towards an area of their choice; for example a cause with personal significance (cancer, multiple sclerosis, etc.).

2. Funds can be directed to causes that would not be necessarily of great interest on a nationwide basis (for example cures for rare conditions).

3. Causes are handled by teams that are dedicated to that cause; this leads to more targeted advertising and awareness campaigns.

4. Greater transparency as funds are handled by a team that has a single purpose as opposed to taxation proceeds which are all lumped before being redistributed.

5. Charities are answerable to their donors and therefore have an incentive to minimise costs and wastage. This increases trust.

6. Different charities may choose to concentrate on different aspects of a particular cause or may approach the same problems in different ways. Such diversity is more constructive than a single-handed governmental approach.

7. Charities are better able to find innovative solutions to find new sources of funds and to address problems at local level.

8. Charities may be better able to highlight important issues that need to be addressed and to raise government awareness.

9. Small charities may spend a large proportion of their funds on overheads and therefore may only allocate a small proportion of their revenue to the causes they deal with.

10. Several charities may deal with the same cause, thus leading to duplication of effort and overheads.

Consequences of leaving decisions to the government

1. Funds would most likely be directed to areas that affect the greatest number of people. It could thus be argued that the money would be used in the best interest of society as a whole rather than small numbers of individuals.

2. Government would be able to pool resources (e.g. advertising) thus reducing overheads and general costs.

3. Government would collect funds through taxation rather than donations. This would effectively force every taxpayer to contribute towards all causes rather than leaving it to individual choice. Higher taxes may build resentment.

4. Government may choose to allocate funds only to causes affecting large numbers of people or to causes that have a strong lobby group. This would act against the smaller causes.

5. Government may choose to exploit the allocation of charitable funds for political aims. For example, increasing funding towards arthritis sufferers 6 months before an election would undoubtedly secure an important proportion of the elderly vote.

Discussion

In practice, charities (particularly the bigger institutions) are partly funded by government and partly by the public. In particular, charities are often best placed to decide which research is needed to solve a particular problem and they are, in a sense, entrusted by the government to make the right decision. Such a system enables a good combination of general governmental intervention towards causes that are of national interest, while enabling individuals to contribute to causes that matter to them at a personal level. Therefore the answer to the question does not have to be black and white as both can cohabit quite happily.

10.23 What are the advantages and disadvantages of admitting when mistakes are made?

This question not only tests your integrity, but also your understanding of why integrity matters. The question looks very theoretical, calling for a list that you could simply learn and regurgitate; however, obviously, many candidates will come up with a similar list and you therefore need to distinguish yourself from the rest by bringing your personal experiences into your answer.

Advantages of admitting when mistakes are made

1. You are able to repair the mistake much more quickly because you can involve others in the process.

2. You can openly identify areas of possible improvement and gain support from your superiors to deal with them.

3. You may originally annoy people but they would be grateful for your honesty. In the long term, owning up to your mistakes may encourage people to trust you more because they know that you are honest.

4. If you admit the mistake and apologise early enough, the matter is much more likely to be resolved without such drastic consequences.

Disadvantages of admitting when mistakes are made

1. Your colleagues and patients may lower their opinion of you.

2. You may be sacked, sued, struck off, or all of the aforementioned.

3. Patients may lose trust towards you and/or the medical profession.

Bringing examples into your answer

It is crucial that you mention examples in order to make your answer more personal and more interesting; otherwise it will resemble everyone else's answer. When you give examples, keep your descriptions to two or three sentences.

Here are a few effective (partial) examples:

… Admitting a mistake straight away may help you maintain good relationships with others as well as their trust. For example, last summer I was manning the till at a clothes shop and forgot to give the client a discount to which she was entitled to and had alluded to. She had said nothing at the time, but as she was walking out of the shop, I realised my mistake and ran to catch up with her and inform her of the mistake. The client was then given some money back. Afterwards she told me that she had noticed the mistake but hadn't dared coming back to ask for her money. She thanked me for my efforts and said that she appreciated the honesty…

… Three months ago, I was asked to write an article for the school's newsletter and had been given a deadline of 30 May. Unfortunately I had entered it into my diary as 30 June and only realised my mistake 3 days before the deadline. Rather than rush the writing of the article, I contacted the editor to apologise for my oversight, gave him a truthful explanation and he agreed to extend the deadline by 3 days to give me more time to write the piece. He actually also apologised himself for not issuing reminders earlier…

… A possible disadvantage of owning up to your mistakes is that you might lose some trust from others. During my Duke of Edinburgh expedition, I sent the team down the wrong track. In the end, that mistake had no serious consequences in that it only lengthened the walk by about 10 minutes. In view of the fact that we had reached the correct destination within the correct timeframe I could have kept quiet about it, but I thought that it would be best to own up to it. The next day, I was banned by the team leader from looking at the map because he felt that I might make another mistake. I did argue that I had reflected on my mistake and understood where I had gone wrong, but to no avail.

10.24	**Do you think it is right for doctors to have conferences, training sessions and study material sponsored by pharmaceutical companies or other corporate sponsors?**

You need to balance professional integrity against the need for education, which may not be provided if such sponsorship did not exist.

Advantages of allowing corporate sponsorship

1. Education budgets are small and many doctors must pay for their education out of their own pocket. This acts as a deterrent and enabling corporate sponsorship allows doctors to develop faster.
2. Gives doctors greater awareness of courses available through circulars sent by corporate sponsors.
3. Allows good introduction to new products from pharmaceutical companies.
4. Allows greater relationship building with the industry.

Disadvantages of allowing corporate sponsorship

1. Sponsors might only support speakers who are biased in their favour (risk of corruption, however small).
2. Doctors may feel obliged to prescribe certain drugs rather than others as a result.

Discussion

Although there is a risk of bias associated with such sponsorship (and the risk must be real, otherwise the companies would not provide funding!), ultimately you must balance this against the need for education. It is simply a matter of being conscious of the risks involved and of making sure that you are not unduly influenced.

Obviously, this will also depend on the nature of the gift. For example, a cheque for £150 to attend a conference based in London would not cause a real problem. But what about an all-expenses paid one-week trip to Barbados for a conference sponsored by a major pharmaceutical? The answer would very much depend on the nature of the work you will be doing there. It is also generally accepted that the gift should be limited to the doctor himself and that no sponsorship should be allowed for travelling spouses (as it would obviously serve no educational purpose).

10.25	**Do you think it is appropriate for doctors to accept small gifts from patients as a thank you gesture?**

There are two aspects to consider:

1 – Professional judgement. As a doctor, you must care for all patients without prejudice, i.e. you cannot be influenced by other factors, and certainly not bribes. The question now is: does a small thank you gesture represent a bribe or not? Is it likely to influence your judgement? What if it were a gift with a higher value? Where is the limit?

2 – Doctor-Patient relationship. What if the present comes from an old lady whom you have been treating for many years and who is obviously not trying to bribe you? What would be the impact on the doctor-patient relationship of refusing the gift?

To bring a successful resolution to the problem, you will need to exercise your professional judgement without endangering your relationship with the patient.

Discussion

Essentially, the main problem associated with accepting the gift is whether you will be influenced by it. If the gift were a box of chocolates, one could barely argue that you would treat a patient better as a result of that gift. But if it were £500 in cash, then you may be influenced, even if subconsciously. Or, even worse, the patient could use this as a weapon later on when they do need you. Many Trusts have adopted policies to deal with this. Policies vary, but generally are as follows:

Policy 1: Accept nothing. If you really cannot refuse it because you fear that it would endanger the doctor-patient relationship (e.g. an old granny's box of chocolates), there are a number of options open to you which would enable you not to benefit directly from the gift:

- Share with staff or other patients (if it can be shared: chocolates for example)
- Give to charity (particularly if it is cash) or place the money in the practice's fund to be used to improve services (e.g. artwork, repaint the waiting room, etc.)

Policy 2: Accept if small gift in kind (e.g. flowers, small pen, chocolates) but do not accept cash. If the value of the item is over a certain amount (say £10) then discuss with practice manager. The advantage of such policy is that you can accept small gifts and therefore avoid damaging the doctor-patient relationship for most situations. If the gift is too great, discussing with the manager ensures that others are aware of the situation and that you are not abusing the situation.

Policy 3: Tiered approach. Below a small amount (say £10), accept. Between that amount and a medium amount (say £10 to £30), discuss with practice manager. Above the medium amount (£30), refuse.

How to handle it
Your first step would be to familiarise yourself with the procedures in your practice or hospital so that you know how to handle the matter. If there is no policy, you will need to look at the level of the gift and the intent behind the gift. For example, there will be no real harm in accepting a small bouquet of flowers from a long-term patient, but it may look odd to accept an expensive case of wine from a relatively new patient.

Generally speaking, if you have any doubt about what to do, there is no harm in raising the issue with a manager or a senior colleague. They will appreciate your openness and integrity.

You must also ensure that you communicate adequately with the patient, particularly if you are going to refuse the gift. It should be explained clearly and politely that you appreciate their gift but that it could be seen as clouding your judgement.

Typical probing questions

Once you have answered the question about the small gift, interviewers tend to like asking about all sorts of gifts. Regular appearances include:

▪ **What if you receive a cauliflower?** (Yes it was a real question!) Unless this is a rare breed that you do not yet have in your collection, you are unlikely to be influenced by such a gift. There are therefore virtually no risks of possible influence here. (You may wonder about the patient's mental state though!)

- **What if the gift is only £2 in cash?** The gift is small so the risk is minimal, but the fact that it is cash means that you should really avoid keeping it. Give it to charity or to the practice's/ward's funds.

- **What if the patient gives you a bottle of wine every year?** You need to see how this fits with the relationship that you have with the patient. If you manage their chronic condition all year round, then the gift is merely a thank you present with no real other intent. If, however, you only see the patient once every 5 years for a fungal infection, you would wonder about the reasons behind the gift. Discussing the situation with a senior colleague would help you sort it out promptly and professionally.

Candidates are usually scared of such questions because interviewers can ask them in many different formats. However, if you always go back to first principles, you have little chance of getting it wrong. Always explain the principles behind your reasoning.

10.26	You are the Health Secretary and you have a budget of £10m available to you every year. With that budget, you will be able to make a treatment or procedure available on the NHS. You have been given the choice between only two options: a treatment that will considerably alleviate the pain of arthritis sufferers and a surgical procedure designed to repair a hole in the heart of neonates. Both treatments/procedures have exactly the same overall annual cost. What would you do?

Since, for the purpose of this question, you are the Health Secretary and not a doctor, you do not have to stick firmly to the established ethical principles, although using them as a guide will be useful in helping you establish an answer to the question. Obviously, dealing with this issue at a macro level, your main concern will be to obtain the best value for money from the point of view of society as a whole.

Benefit to the individual

One issue that you need to consider is the effect that each treatment is likely to have on the individuals that will receive it.

- Arthritis sufferers will experience a better quality of life. They may be able to regain a degree of physical ability that they had long lost. There may also be other treatments available, even if they are slightly less effective.

- For the neonates, it is simply a case of life or death. If they do not get the treatment on the NHS, they will need to obtain it privately at great cost, which is likely to be prohibitive.

From the point of view of the individual, it could therefore be argued that the neonates will clearly benefit most as it will enable them to live, while arthritis sufferers will simply benefit from an enhanced quality of life.

Benefit to society

There are many ways in which society will be affected by the decision:

- How many people are affected? If there was a large discrepancy between the number of people affected by the treatment every year (e.g.

if the £10m budget can provide treatment for only two neonates versus 1 million arthritis sufferers) then you would need to give careful consideration to the question.

- How much will those affected contribute to society? For example, the neonates will go on to lead normal lives that would be taken away from them if they did not get the treatment. On the other hand, those with arthritis (who may be young as well as old) could take up better jobs and increase their contribution to society. Those who had to stop work because of the arthritis may be able to start work and lead a "normal" life again. The answer to this would depend on the effectiveness of the drug, and the occupations of those involved as well as their average age.

- How much aftercare will be needed for the neonates? Does the £10m cater for the whole of their care or simply the initial procedure? The answer may influence the overall cost and therefore the outcome.

Ultimately, there is no answer to this question. It is purely a matter of deciding which arguments you feel are stronger than the others.

Also not to be forgotten: the question is asking you to place yourself in the skin of a politician and any decision may also depend on which alternative is the biggest vote winner. Do you play the sympathy card by choosing in favour of the neonates or do you seek to please arthritis sufferers, most of whom are of voting age? There is no need to be cynical at the interview, though you might want to introduce an air of realism by demonstrating an understanding of the fact that clinical and political decisions are not always based on the same principles.

10.27 Do you think it is right for patients to make the choice as to what is in their own best interest?

Arguments in favour of giving patients the choice

1. Patients are responsible for their own body. If they can make decisions about their lifestyle, they should also be able to make decisions about the healthcare that supports it. They are also more likely to go through with the treatment if they have been involved in the decision making process.

2. Having to explain different options to a patient encourages doctors to take a more thorough approach rather than rushing into their own preferred option. By questioning doctors, patients act as a counterweight and ensure the provision of safer care.

3. Several approaches may be suitable, each with different impacts on the patient's lifestyle. The patient should be able to choose what suits him best.

4. The patient and the doctor share the responsibility for the outcome should anything go wrong.

Arguments against giving patients the choice

1. The patient may not have the background knowledge to make the best decision for themselves.

2. The patient may be unduly influenced by other parties such as relatives.

3. Patients may make decisions based on external information (anecdotes from friends, information from the internet), which may not be accurate or appropriate for their situation.

10.28 People are living longer. Should doctors take credit for it?

Yes, doctors should take credit for it

1. Medical advancement is a key factor in increased longevity. Some diseases are much more easily managed than before and, in some cases such as HIV, are no longer fatal if well managed.

2. Doctors play an important role in educating patients on how to lead healthier lifestyles and provide means of acting on unhealthy behaviours (e.g. smoking cessation, dietary advice, etc.).

No, doctors can't take credit for it (or at least not all of it)

1. Medical advancement is not always credited to doctors. Biochemists and other research-focused professions often play a major role.

2. Doctors are not the only health professionals looking after patients. For example, a patient may be followed up by a nurse once he has seen a doctor (or may even only be seen by a nurse in the first place). In many ways, nurses have closer and more frequent contact with patients and may raise issues that need investigating.

3. Health promotion is not undertaken solely by doctors. School teachers, charities and other organisations also play a vital role.

4. Patients are also more educated because they have easier access to information (e.g. through the internet). They may therefore act upon problems earlier than they would normally have done previously.

10.29 Should doctors have a role in regulating contact sports such as boxing?

Since the question is asking for your opinion, you will need to present both sides of the argument. In this particular case, the balance of argument is clearly in favour of a "Yes" answer, which should make it easier not to sit on the fence (note that the question is not about whether you agree that boxing should be allowed in the first place, but about the involvement of doctors in its regulation).

Arguments against

- Doctors should not be seen to be condoning any behaviour that could negatively affect somebody's health (and in some cases may seriously damage them or even kill them).

Arguments for

- Doctors should be non-judgemental. In the same way that the public does not expect to be judged and patronised with regard to other behaviours such as eating habits and other personal choices, doctors should be able to approach the issue of boxing in a constructive manner.

- Not getting involved would actually be worse than getting involved. Boxing will take place whether doctors like it or not. By helping to regulate the sport, doctors can actually influence the way the sport functions. This is consistent with the principle of beneficence (see Section 5.8).

- Boxing is primarily attracting a more deprived portion of the population. That population is generally hard to reach, as a result of which it suffers greater health problems. Involving doctors at that level may give an opportunity to promote other messages about healthy living.

10.30 Should doctors show a good example to patients?

Arguments in favour of doctors showing a good example

- Doctors need credibility in order to be trusted by their patients. A patient may find it difficult to take seriously a recommendation to stop smoking and to eat healthily if he sees his doctor smoking while eating a burger.

Arguments against doctors showing a good example

- This is an issue of individual choice. The health messages given by doctors are commonly accepted facts; it is then down to each individual to treat that advice in the way they want.

- Defining "good example" is not easy. A pattern of behaviour may be a good example for someone and a bad example for someone else. For example, a GP drinking 15 units of alcohol per week would be a good example for most people, but not for an ex-alcoholic. In addition, people's bodies react differently to others. Some people may have a metabolism that can cope with a certain amount of unhealthy food, while others are more sensitive.

- Following every single health message to the letter with a view to showing a good example may make the doctor's life hell. Which type of food has no sugar, no salt, no fat, and can still taste interesting?

What matters is that everyone should do everything in moderation. Unfortunately, it does not matter if you eat burgers in moderation. The day a patient sees you eating one, he will assume that it is part of your normal diet. This is a dilemma that will never be resolved until patients are able to take personal responsibility for their own health.

10.31	60% of medical school applicants are female. Why do you think that is?

No one really knows the real reason, and there are probably several factors that come into play. You will therefore be judged on your ability to display a range of possible reasons and on the clarity of your reasoning.

- **Statistics:** there are more girls than boys alive at the age of 17 anyway for several reasons including the fact that more girls than boys are born and that boys experience a higher mortality than girls during their teenage years due to risk taking.

- **Academic success:** girls tend to perform better than boys at exams, achieving better grades. They may also feel that they can resist the pressures of medical school better than boys.

- **Government campaigns:** for a long time, Medicine was a male-dominated profession and the government campaigned hard to encourage girls to take up the profession. This may have led to an increase in applications through the influence of school teachers.

- **Work-life balance:** Medicine has changed dramatically. A general awareness of the stress levels experienced by doctors together with the introduction of the European Working Time Directive has helped reduce working hours. In addition, numerous posts have been created for flexible trainees and workers. This makes it easier for women who want to have a family to pursue a career at the same time. The most dramatic effect has been for GPs.

- **Type of work:** women may feel more at ease in building a good rapport with patients. Also, boys may be more inclined to take up jobs that pay more (more money or prestige driven), such as law and finance.

10.32	What are the advantages and disadvantages of the increasing role of nurses?

Your answer to this question should be diplomatic. This is a controversial issue on which many doctors hold very strong views. At the interview, your job is not to get into this controversy but to debate the advantages and disadvantages. Also, don't forget that nurses may be on the panel. Be careful not to upset them!

Advantages

1. It may free up doctors' time, which enables doctors to concentrate on more complex patients or procedures. In turn, this reduces waiting lists and therefore increases patient satisfaction.

2. It can provide better continuity of care for patients. Doctors change posts often throughout their training whereas nurses do not move on as frequently.

3. Nurses may be able to spend more time with patients. This also increases patient satisfaction and may help identify other issues that could not be identified in a short consultation time (e.g. psychosocial issues).

4. It acts as a motivator for nurses, who can now have careers well beyond the basic nursing level. This encourages retention of staff, motivation and good morale.

5. It may be more cost-effective. However, some studies have shown that in fact the savings are not noticeable or that nurses may actually prove more expensive. Although most nurses (not all!) do get paid less than doctors, they may see patients for a longer period of time and, if they cannot deal with a patient, they will still refer them to the doctor (when it may have been more cost-effective for the patient to see the doctor in the first place).

Disadvantages

1. Nurses are taken away from frontline nursing care (though admittedly only a small number of nurses are affected by this).

2. Nurses take charge of less complex patients and simple procedures, which were traditionally dealt with by junior doctors. This will therefore reduce the opportunities for junior doctors to encounter these patients and procedures, which will impact on their training.

3. Nurses with extended roles work on a protocol basis. Their input is therefore limited to the boundaries of the protocol. In addition, since the nurses' training is not as comprehensive as the doctors', they may not be able to recognise at all times when a patient should be handled outside the protocol.

4. There is an issue of patients' confidence. Patients may not want to be treated by nurses and may request that a qualified doctor deals with them instead.

To finish on a positive note, it would be good to explain how, ultimately, it is all about finding the right balance so that doctors and nurses can share duties but in a way that works best for patients (who should be everyone's first priority).

10.33	Why do people on aeroplanes suffer from Deep Vein Thrombosis from being still in one position, yet this doesn't affect people when they are asleep despite being in the same position for hours?

Deep vein thrombosis (DVT) is a blood clot that forms in a deep leg vein. The deep veins are blood vessels that go through the calf and thigh muscles (i.e. not those you can see just below the skin).

Tip: if at an interview you are asked a question relating to a topic you know little about, ask the interviewers to provide clarification. To answer this question well, you don't need to be an expert on DVT but you need to understand roughly what it is. It is better to ask and provide a sensible answer, than gamble and give a half-baked answer. In this particular case, they are not testing your medical knowledge but your lateral thinking capabilities.

List of possible reasons include:

- DVT is often caused by inactivity (hence why, when you fly, airlines recommend that you should move around the plane to stretch your legs). When you sleep, you change position during the night whereas when you fly you are often confined to a small space, making it hard to move sufficiently.

- Reduced cabin pressure, reduced oxygen levels in the plane, dehydration caused by not drinking much water, and drinking too much alcohol (often freely available) might also be possible causes. When you sleep, you may get dehydrated too, but people may find it easier to get up and help themselves to a glass of water. None of these have been proven yet to be actual causes, but they are all being researched. They are also all causes that someone without knowledge may intuitively think about and therefore mentioning them would show the interviewers that you are able to come up with sensible ideas.

| **10.34** | **The time that it takes to become a consultant has been decreased. What are the implications of this?** |

This question requires no knowledge of the training pathway for consultants (see Section 5.3 if you want detail on that), only logic and lateral thinking.

Possible implications include:

- The same amount of knowledge may need to be crammed into a shorter period, leading to a more superficial learning process. Putting it simply, new consultants may not be as knowledgeable as old consultants. One could argue, however, that this is counterbalanced by a more efficient training programme (in other words, the old consultants may have wasted some time during their training, making it unnecessarily longer).

- In view of the decreased amount of time, consultants may not be able to train in all aspects of their chosen specialty, and may need to sub-specialise early on. For example, whereas beforehand an orthopaedic surgeon would train to handle all aspects of orthopaedic surgery first and then choose a sub-specialty later, it may no longer be possible to offer such breadth of training at the start. Consequently, rather than become an all-encompassing orthopaedic surgeon, a trainee may have to specialise straight away in hip and knee surgery and nothing else. This would produce much more specialised surgeons, but may also cause problems when doing on-call duties as new consultants would not necessarily have the knowledge and ability to deal with every problem they may face.

- In the short term there will be a sharp increase in the number of consultants. If this is matched by an availability of posts then this will lead to a more consultant-delivered service; if not, this will lead to more unemployment amongst qualified doctors.

10.35 Do you think a doctor's enthusiasm wanes over time?

As with all questions asking for an opinion or a debate, you need to weigh both sides of the argument. In this case, the answer is unlikely to be a clear-cut answer of the type "No, because Medicine is so exciting" or "Yes, everything can be boring in time". Your answer should therefore seek to explain which factors may lead doctors to lose some enthusiasm whilst also painting a picture that is not apocalyptic.

In other words, the gist of your answer should be "Of course, one cannot always retain the same level of enthusiasm throughout any period of time and there are issues which may make doctors' enthusiasm wane; but in many cases, these would be balanced by the more positive sides of the profession."

You should also use your answer to demonstrate that you understand the pros and cons of working in Medicine (see Q.7.11) and to talk about your work experience and your own personal attributes.

Example of an effective answer

On the whole, it is always very hard to stay enthusiastic for anything without working at it. For example, a couple of years ago, I was part of a debating society and, though it was very enjoyable at first, it soon became routine and there was a real danger that attending the debates would soon become a chore. I addressed that by getting more involved in organising the debates and taking on responsibilities, which gave me more variety and therefore more enjoyment.

The same would apply to Medicine. At first, you enjoy seeing patients, you learn all the time, you discover a new point every day. As doctors become more experienced they might start to fall into a routine (for example, doing clinics or attend theatre every day), which could lead to a degree of despondency. Some might address that by taking on new roles (for example, teaching, or management roles), whilst others might just let it happen. Having said that, those who take on new roles might feel that they are becoming more and more distant from patient care, and may become disillusioned at the fact that their role is no longer that of a traditional doctor.

On top of the routine element, there are features of the medical profession that could encourage doctors to lose their enthusiasm, for example a prolonged exposure to difficult patients, political interference and the feeling that you cannot control the system, etc.

As a future doctor, I am sure that I will meet situations where I will lose my enthusiasm for a variety of things. It is a natural human feeling. However, being a natural optimist and a very proactive person, I am sure that those times would only be temporary and that, were I ever to feel despondent, I would know how to deal with it and would be re-energised by the thought that I am there to help others.

Another example of an effective answer

Whenever you do something for a long time, there are bound to be good times as well as bad times. For example, I am sure that there are doctors who have the feeling that their job has become routine or is not what they thought it would be, perhaps because they have become involved too much in activities which they do not enjoy (such as management) or because they spend a lot of their time dealing with the same problems, or because they meet a lot of patients who are uncooperative. When you study Medicine, you tend to be exposed for short periods of time to a lot of specialties and that can be very exciting. After that, learning to become a specialist can also be very exciting because you are constantly accumulating new knowledge, seeing increasingly complex patients and learning your craft. So when you have come through that stage, there may come a time when you reach a plateau – some sort of mid-life crisis – causing your enthusiasm to wane.

Having said that, I am also sure that there are doctors who become more enthusiastic as they become more specialised and feel more in control. Some doctors might also rather enjoy the opportunity to take on different roles in teaching, research or management, and use those roles as a means to keep their medical career interesting.

For my part, I have always enjoyed taking on new challenges and new roles – for example I have been involved in activities as diverse as teaching local children maths in my spare time or organising social activities for my school. So I am sure I will be able to ensure that I build a career path which keeps me interested.

10.36 What could be the implications of medical advancement on medical training?

Medical advancement means that the volume of information increases constantly. This could lead to increased training time. If we want to avoid lengthening the training to cover that extra ground then new, more effective and more efficient methods of training must be found. One way in which this is achieved is by training doctors on core skills first and then allowing them to go on fellowships dealing with areas of interest.

An alternative would be to superspecialise doctors early on so that they only learn a partial section of their specialty. So for example, an orthopaedics surgeon would not train in all aspects of orthopaedics before specialising in hips and knees. Instead he would learn about hips and knees without worrying about anything else. This approach has been tried in the past with limited success. The main problem was that those who had specialised early were only able to handle cases from the limited field in which they had trained. That meant that they could not deal with on calls, nights and weekends, where all-rounders were needed to be able to handle whatever type of problem came through the door.

Medical advancement also means that some tasks can be done more systematically by other people. For example, in the distant past, doctors used to analyse blood or other samples with microscopes, whilst nowadays this will be done either by nurses or a separate pathology lab, leaving doctors to concentrate on more complex activities. As activities are delegated to others, doctors run the risk of being less exposed to some of the basics of Medicine, leaving gaps in their knowledge.

Medical advancement has led to a better understanding of the mechanics and chemistry of the human body, enabling good simulation tools to be built, making training easier.

10.37 Is it best for a doctor to be a good clinician or a good communicator?

The answer to this question is that you need to be both.

Being a good clinician would mean that you are good at diagnosing conditions, excellent at performing procedures and good at setting out effective management plans for patients. However, although this looks sufficient on the surface, none of that can be done without also being a good communicator. In particular:

- A doctor has to be a good listener. Doctors can't diagnose a condition without getting information from their patients. If they do not engage with patients, patients may not tell the doctor what he needs to know. Being a good listener also means that doctors are able to read between the lines and pick up information from a patient's body language and general attitude. A doctor who does not listen may miss the fact that a patient has reservations about a particular course of treatment. Doctors also need to be attentive to and listen to their staff. Doctors will need information from the whole team in order to make decisions.

- A doctor needs to be good at communicating information to patients in a way that the patient can understand it. Different patients have different levels of understanding, different cultural backgrounds and different attitudes towards their condition. Talking to a child, a middle-aged adult or a senile person requires different sets of skills. A doctor also needs to communicate well with his team, giving clear instructions, and keeping clear notes.

- Doctors need to be good at handling conflict and negotiating solutions with both patients and colleagues. Dealing with a demanding or an angry patient requires a lot of tact and an appropriate tone of voice. Similarly, when in conflict with other colleagues, doctors need to be respectful and, whilst ensuring they resolve their differences, they need to ensure they maintain good relationships with everyone. This requires good negotiation and influencing skills.

In your answer, try to illustrate your points with anecdotes from your work experience.

10.38 Which question would you most want to ask if you were interviewing others to enter medical school?

The basis for this question is really to determine what you feel you should find out about a prospective doctor and basically if you have any common sense.

Essentially, what you will want to know is whether the candidate is capable of going through medical school and capable of becoming a good doctor. The question you would most want to ask would therefore need to be fairly broad-ranging to allow the candidate to express himself about himself. In that respect, any question you would ask would revolve around the themes of motivation, ambition and interpersonal skills. For example:

- Tell me about yourself
- What can you offer to our school?
- What are your main strengths?
- Why should we choose you?
- Why are you the best candidate?
- Why do you think you will make a good doctor? etc.

These are questions of a similar nature that enable you to detect what a person feels they have to offer and how they organise information. To an extent, these questions also enable you to see how much preparation the candidate has done on a topic that they should know more about than anyone else: themselves.

- Why do you want to do Medicine?
- Where do you see yourself in 10 years' time?
- What are you seeking to achieve in your medical career?

These questions are motivation questions that also allow the candidate to express and demonstrate a variety of skills.

Of course, there are many other questions that you can ask and this book will provide you with a wide range. It almost does not matter which question you choose providing you are able to explain what you are seeking to achieve by asking it. You should also describe what type of answer the candidate would need to give to convince you that they are suitable.

Make sure that you are able to answer your own favourite question!

Example of an effective answer

The question that I would most want to ask would be a question that is not too direct and gives the candidate a good opportunity to talk about their multiple facets while giving me information about their motivation for Medicine, their interpersonal skills, their ambitions and their organisational skills. The question would therefore need to be a general background question such as "Tell me about yourself", or "Why do you think you can cope with medical school?" Through these questions I would expect the candidate to present a wide range of information in an organised and easily digestible format, which would include:

- A general academic background

- A description of his work experience, what he observed and gained personally from it

- An idea of why he feels that Medicine is the career that he wishes to pursue

- An interest in research and teaching others

- His listening abilities and empathy as well as his ability to work well in teams and lead them when required

- An ability to make decisions

- A hard-working temperament, an ability to work well under pressure and a recognition that having a social life and hobbies is important to help anticipate stress and deal with it.

10.39 A long distance lorry driver has just been diagnosed with diabetes, which he needs to control with daily injections of insulin (at least two per day). He will also be required to maintain a low sugar diet.

His wife is not working; they have three children under the age of 18, two of whom are at an expensive private school, and a large mortgage.

Driving regulations are such that professional drivers who have insulin-controlled diabetes are required to demonstrate that their condition is under control in order to keep their driving licence otherwise they may lose their licence.

What are the issues that you, as a doctor, may wish to address with the patient?

The text of this question is lengthy and, at an interview, would usually be given to you before you enter the room so that you have time to consider the different layers of information it provides. Make sure you use all the information given to you.

Whenever you have to deal with any patient-related situations, you should consider the following four angles:

1. Physical
2. Psychological
3. Social
4. Financial.

Physical
- The condition requires 2 injections per day. Does he feel that he can achieve it within the constraints of his driving job (bearing in mind that he has no choice otherwise he may lose his licence and therefore his livelihood).

- Maintaining a healthy diet whilst on the road may be hard to achieve (the food available at service stations is not always the healthiest). How does he think he will be able to cope with it? You might recommend that he sees a dietician for advice on how to deal with this problem.

Psychological
- How does he feel about the diagnosis? The fear of losing his job may be daunting for him.

- Has he discussed the situation with his family? How are they supporting him psychologically?

- Does he have friends in similar situations he can talk to?

- Is there an association for lorry drivers that he could contact for support? What about a diabetes charity?

- Is there a risk that he may fall into depression? You may consider referring him to a counsellor.

Social
- Other than psychologically, is his family helping by making sure that they don't eat foods he can't eat in front of him or by sharing some elements of his healthier diet?

Financial
- He seems to have a lot of large expenses and is the main bread winner. Has he discussed with his family the consequences of not being able to manage his condition, i.e. of losing his licence?

- Does he have alternative ways of earning a living? Would his wife be able to work?

- Has he considered the possibility of taking his children out of private education? Has he talked to them about the prospect?

You may encounter such scenarios in any interview. The main issue here is to make sure that you look at the whole picture and not simply the medical side of the problem. Medicine is not just about taking medication or doing procedures according to given protocols. It is about taking a patient-centred approach, which includes dealing with psychosocial issues as well. The interviewers will therefore be very keen to ensure that they recruit candidates who are able to think more laterally about all the relevant issues.

10.40 For religious reasons, Jehovah's Witnesses cannot accept blood transfusions. Would you be happy to let a Jehovah's Witness die because he refused a blood transfusion?

There are several aspects to consider:

Patient's autonomy. Jehovah's Witnesses do not accept the use of blood products from another person even if such a decision may lead to death. In accordance with the principle of autonomy, any patient is entitled to make their own decision, even if this defies the doctor's idea of their best interest. Therefore, if the patient is competent, or if they have made a "living will" refusing a transfusion, then you will have to respect their decision.

Beneficence. As a doctor, you still have a duty of beneficence, even if it is sometimes overridden by the patient's autonomy. Without exercising undue pressure, you must make sure that they have made their decision with full knowledge of all the facts and that they understand the consequences of not accepting the transfusion. There are also other aspects that you may want to consider. For example, is transfusion the only option? Are there other people that the patient can talk to before making a final decision (for example, a liaison group for Jehovah's Witnesses)? Once you have done everything you can for the patient, you can only accept their final verdict. It does not mean that you will be happy to let them die. In a sense, you may take it as a personal failure, but you should be content with the thought that you have tried your absolute best.

Competence/Capacity. Just because someone makes a decision that you feel is irrational (e.g. accepting to die by refusing treatment), it does not mean that they are not competent to make that decision. If you felt that someone was making an irrational decision because they may not be competent, you would need to seek advice from colleagues and possibly a psychiatrist about the way forward. If the patient were deemed to be non-competent, you would still need to take account of their beliefs and what they would have decided if they had been competent. You may need help from the relatives for that.

10.41 What would you do if a known Jehovah's Witness arrived in A&E unconscious, bleeding profusely and needing an urgent blood transfusion?

The first thing you would do is stop the bleeding. Unless the patient had previously indicated that they would not want to be treated in case of an emergency, nothing would prevent you from doing it because the patient is unconscious and cannot give consent (hence you would need to act in their best interest).

The issue of the transfusion is a bit more delicate. First of all, you should not jump to conclusions. The patient may be a Jehovah's Witness but they may not follow their religion in an orthodox manner. Thus you cannot assume that the patient would be against a transfusion unless they had made a specific request not to be transfused. Such a request could be either documented in your notes if the patient had been in hospital previously, or they may even carry a card with them. If you have any doubts, your first port of call would be to see if you have quick access to a relative. They may be present or easily reachable. They may assist you in deciding what the patient would have wanted, had they been able to make an informed decision. Note that, although the relatives can assist you in the decision, the final decision rests with you.

If you have no information about what the patient would have wanted, or if time is of the essence (the question says the patient needs an urgent transfusion), you will need to act in what you believe to be the best interest of the patient. To play it safe, you may wish to investigate any alternative to blood transfusion. Alternatively, you may simply decide to go ahead with the transfusion. In doing so, you may be taking the risk that the patient may later disagree with your approach and take legal action but provided you can justify your decision, you have nothing to fear. For this reason, you may want to involve seniors and other members of your team at an early stage, including perhaps the hospital's legal team to cover all sides.

10.42	A mother comes to A&E with a child who is bleeding pro-fusely and refuses to allow you to administer a blood trans-fusion to the child. Why do you think this may be and what would you do?

Make sure you do not fall into the trap. Everyone has heard about Jehovah's Witnesses refusing blood transfusion and this is an easy link to make. You should open your mind to other possibilities. Aside from religious beliefs, it is also possible that the mother is simply worried about the procedure itself. This could be because of the thought of having someone else's blood in her own child or because she fears a risk of infection (e.g. HIV, Hepatitis or other infection). Once you have addressed the bleeding, you will need to address with the mother the reasons why she is unwilling to give consent for the transfusion. Depending on the reasons, you would act in different ways.

If the child is deemed to be competent (see Section 5.10), then you can accept consent from the child himself. Although you would need to manage the communication process with the mother (who may be angry at your decision), you would be entitled to disregard her opinion. Once the (competent) child has given his consent, you would simply proceed with the necessary treatment.

For the remainder of this question, we will assume that the child is not competent, in which case consent for the procedure would need to be obtained from the mother herself.

If the mother is simply worried about the act of the transfusion, the risk of infection or other practical issues, then it is more a matter of reassuring her with a suitable level of listening skills and empathy, as well as explaining to her how blood is screened and how safe the blood would be for the child. You may want to involve other people in the discussion such as a senior colleague (some patients react better to consultants than to junior doctors), a nurse or anyone the patient would trust. With sufficient explanation, the mother may then change her views and concur with your line of treatment.

If the mother still refuses treatment, either by principle alone or because of an underlying religious belief, then the decision to treat would have to be taken in line with what you believe to be in the best interest of the child. If you do treat (going against parental decision), the approach would be different depending on whether this is an emergency or not. If it is an emergency (i.e. you need to give blood straight away), you would need to be sure that, should criminal proceedings be taken against you at a later date, you are confident that you can defend your actions as being taken in the best interest of the patient. If the treatment does not need to be administered immediately, then there is an opportunity to discuss the situation further with your multidisciplinary team and, in rare circumstances, to apply for a court order which would allow you to proceed with the treatment.

In any case, you will always need to ensure that you involve senior or specially trained colleagues in the discussions as much as you can, as well as the hospital's legal team if there is time for this and if there is any risk of the matter leading to litigation.

10.43 You have one liver available for transplant and must choose one of two possible patients on the transplant list. One is an ex-alcoholic mother with two young children and the other one is a 13-year-old child with a congenital (from birth) liver defect. They both have equal clinical needs. How would you go about choosing who gets the liver?

This is a very common question, which comes in different forms. You sometimes also see the issue of smokers and lung transplants. You must remember that there is no clear-cut answer to such a question. There are only issues to raise. Also note that the question is not actually "Who would you give the liver to?" but "How would you go about choosing?" The panel is far more interested in your thought process than in whether you can zoom in on a particular answer.

Prejudice and assumptions

There are a number of traps that candidates fall into because they adopt an approach that is too simplistic. Look at the following statements made by candidates to justify their choice and try to derive why they may not be entirely suitable:

- The 13-year-old girl is younger than the mother and therefore will live longer and has more to offer to society.

- The mother is an alcoholic and therefore her problem is self-inflicted. That makes the young girl more deserving.

- Most alcoholics relapse. Therefore the liver will be wasted on the mother. She will just start drinking again.

- If the mother dies, the two children may find it hard to cope without her. This would be unfair to them and therefore the mother needs to be given the liver.

The common thread between all these statements is that they are making some kind of assumption. Although there may be some truth behind those assumptions and therefore they cannot be completely discounted, it is dangerous to take such a simplistic approach. You should recognise that the information available in the question is simply not sufficient to make any kind of decision. In your answer, you should highlight specific additional information that would help you justify these assumptions. The following considerations should give you a framework of how to think through this.

Ethical considerations – how to approach the question

When dealing with ethical situations, you must take a step back and identify the main issues that the question raises. Do not stick to headline or bold statements as for every bold statement that you make there will be a counter-argument. Instead, you must adopt a structured approach that demonstrates that you can think logically.

In this scenario, we are considering giving a scarce resource to competing patients with equal clinical need. One of the main factors that you will consider is the patients' ability to survive that treatment in the short term as well as in the long term. There are many characteristics of each individual case which go beyond the physical factors, which you can allude to. But again beware of simple speculation and harsh judgements. Factors to consider are as follows:

Biological factors
These are factors that will influence survival of the procedure but also successful grafting and decreased likelihood of rejection.

- **Matching**. An obvious criterion to consider is whether the liver available is a suitable match for the patient both from a tissue type and a size point of view. Although this may sound simple, you should mention this at the start so that you can concentrate on the less obvious matters during your answer.

- **Age**. Although age is not a discriminatory factor on the sole basis of a number (principle of Justice), you will look differently at a situation where a patient who is old is concerned. For example, an older person may be less able to survive surgery or its complications, and therefore may be considered less suitable compared to a younger and fitter person. Having said that, an older person may also be considered fitter than a younger one. This will be dictated by individual circumstances. Doctors often talk about someone's physiological or biological age, rather than the number of years they have actually lived.

303

- **Co-morbidity**. One of the patients may have other diseases that substantially affect their life expectancy, such as some form of terminal cancer with little time to live. In addition, co-morbidities may affect their ability to deal with the long-term medications (immunosuppressants) that they will be required to take after surgery.

- **Risk of recurrence of the underlying disease**. There are diseases that are not cured by removal and simple replacement of an organ. For example, a congenital metabolic defect which leads to the accumulation of a toxin that damages the liver will not be eradicated simply by replacing the liver. Transplant will merely postpone the death of the patient until the new liver becomes damaged too.

In the case of alcoholism, this is a condition which, if it continues, will also affect the new liver and to some extent it falls into the above category. However, it is avoidable, unlike congenital conditions, and therefore may also fall into the next category. See below.

Psychosocial factors
These are factors or issues driven by the individual's surrounding lifestyle, environment and psychological state, but which may ultimately lead to biological reasons for a less successful outcome following transplantation.

A healthy lifestyle will contribute to the individual's overall health and any decision may therefore be influenced by the lifestyle that the patient may follow after transplantation. But please be aware that this should be an objective consideration rather than a prejudiced assumption. For example:

- **Lack of commitment to maintain a lifestyle appropriate to maximise chances of success.** In the case of an alcoholic, this would mean assessing the probability that this particular patient may relapse. However, although it may be true that the majority of alcoholics relapse, her position will need to be assessed individually. Even if she presented a risk of relapse (for example because it was established that she did not have a very strong will, or if she indicated that she would probably drink again), it would not necessarily mean that you would have to give up on her. On the contrary, she would require supplementary care of a psychological or psychiatric nature.

- **Failure to adhere to post-operative long-term immunotherapy and follow-up.** Not taking the required medication would lead to a rejection of the liver, therefore rendering the whole process useless.

Impact on society

The principle of Justice allows for the fact that doctors may choose the good of society above the good of the individual patient. Essentially, you would be looking at the loss to society resulting from the death of that patient. It may be very obvious that the two patients have very different number of quality years to live (e.g. a 2-month-old baby versus a 100-year-old man) but, in most cases, it will not be so clear-cut. However, talking through these issues will help you score valuable points. Some of the issues you could consider include:

▪ Two children may be orphaned, with adverse consequences on their life. They may also need to be supported by the State.

▪ It would not be fair for the young girl to be refused treatment because the other patient had children (after all she never had the chance to have children herself. Also you would not want to encourage people to have children in order to get better care for themselves).

▪ Although two children would be without a mother, it has happened to many people before, who then went on to lead successful lives.

▪ If the young girl were not to receive the transplant, her parents would suffer equally. Those parents may be old and may require her support in years to come.

Overall, as you can see, there are many contradictions that come into the debate and that you will never be able to resolve without further information. The final decision is made not by an individual clinician but as a result of deliberations by a specialist panel of multidisciplinary staff. Your role is to balance the arguments and demonstrate an open mind.

10.44	What would you do if an obese patient demanded an immediate total hip replacement, which will fail in 6 months?

There are several issues to consider here.

Justice (clinical need)

The patient has a clinical need that is the same as other people (who may not be obese) and therefore he is equally entitled to the hip replacement as anyone else. One could also effectively argue that this should be a basic human right for the patient.

Justice (interest of society)

On the other hand, if there is a near certainty that the obesity will make the hip replacement fail, one has to wonder what purpose the hip replacement will serve other than simply relieving the patient for only 6 months to the detriment of other people on whom the money may be spent more efficiently. In other words, there is a risk that the treatment will not really benefit the patient in the long term, and may also go against the interest of society as a whole by diverting resources unnecessarily.

Impact on the patient of going ahead

The patient may actually be worse off in the long run if you went ahead with the operation straight away. The failure may have a psychological impact. In addition, the operation itself presents possible risks of failure, including severe or even fatal complications. In other words, an immediate operation may actually harm the patient, whereas postponing the operation may be more beneficial. This would allow the doctor to fulfil both the beneficence and non-maleficence ethical principles.

Can you do something to resolve the obesity problem before proceeding with the hip replacement?

The main issue here is that the obesity will render the hip replacement useless within a short period of time. If you can work on the obesity and reduce it, then the patient may be able to benefit from a hip replacement but at a later stage. This would involve different steps, including:

- Discussing the nature of the problem with the patient and ensuring that they understand the consequences of the obesity. You will need to work with the patient to achieve a satisfactory outcome.

- Enlisting the help of other professionals such as a dietician and a physiotherapist to guide the patient towards a healthier lifestyle and overcome the pain.

- Ensuring appropriate pain relief for the patient while he is working on the obesity problem.

Providing treatment immediately is not necessarily in the best interest of patients and you must weigh up the different arguments. In this question, you have a perfect opportunity to discuss the various ethical principles and to explain how taking a holistic approach to the care of the patient can actually produce good successful results.

What if the patient insists that he wants the treatment?

Although the patient has a right to autonomy, i.e. to make his own deci-sion, such decisions can only be taken amongst a choice offered to him by the Trust and the doctor. If the Trust has made the decision not to fund hip replacements for any obese patients, then there is little that the patient can do about it and he will need to challenge the Trust's decision in court (as happened in the case of Herceptin). Alternatively, the patient may seek treatment by another Trust that is more willing.

If there are no restrictions imposed by the Trust, the doctor will need to balance the arguments and decide whether the benefits of having the hip replacement outweigh the risks. If the risks outweigh the benefits, the doc-tor could refuse to proceed with the hip replacement. The patient would be entitled to a second opinion from another doctor.

Conclusion: The best approach may therefore be to consider reducing the obesity problem so that the operation can go ahead with fewer risks and a more successful long-term outcome.

10.45	A young woman presents with rheumatoid arthritis. She has tried all the conventional treatments but is still having problems. Unless her symptoms improve, she will have to give up work in the near future. There is a new but very expensive treatment available. Treatment for a single patient costs as much as conventional treatment for ten patients. The drug is not effective in all patients and in some cases gives rise to a worsening of the symptoms. What do you do?

This question gives many clues about the issues to be addressed. Your role will be to highlight those issues and explain the extent to which they present a dilemma.

Beneficence vs. non-maleficence

First, you would need to determine if the treatment would actually benefit or harm the patient based on the patient's history, and your examination and knowledge of the patient. On one hand the drug may go against the patient's best interest by worsening the symptoms, but on the other hand it may improve the symptoms too.

If the balance of probabilities were such that, in your opinion, the patient would be harmed by the new drug then you may consider not prescribing the new drug, even if the patient was asking for it (otherwise you would be going against the non-maleficence principle). If, however, you felt that there was a decent chance that the patient may benefit from the new drug, you would need to discuss the facts with her so that she becomes fully equipped to make a decision as to whether she is prepared to take the risk or not (principle of autonomy). Your role will then consist of providing as much information as possible to help her make that fully informed decision and you would need to ensure that she is not being coerced at any stage.

Impact on society (Justice)

The problem becomes more complex if you introduce the issue of cost and scarce resources into the equation, i.e. if giving the new drug to the patient may actually make others worse off. In your decision-making process, you would need to consider the benefits to the patient versus the benefits to society as a whole. Giving the patient the drug will take valuable resources away from ten other patients, but on the other hand those patients may never materialise. In addition, the impact on society is itself ambiguous. Giving her the drug could have the following impacts:

- **Society will be worse off** because it may open floodgates and many other patients will request the same treatment (in some cases, through court cases). This could prove very expensive indeed, well beyond the ten patients mentioned above. Overall, it may actually divert a vast amount of funds towards a treatment that may or may not work, when those funds may be better utilised in other ways.

- **Society will not benefit.** If the patient does not take the drug then she will need to stop working. Consequently, she will contribute less to society, she is likely to be placed on benefits, she will stop paying taxes and the cost to society may actually be greater than if she were to be placed on the treatment in the first place. She may also have dependants who would be worse off as a result of her decreased level of activity.

The case will need to be judged on its own merits and on personal circumstances at the time. Because of possible financial implications, a decision is likely to involve communications with managers at Trust level to determine whether the treatment may be given.

Such situations are very complex to explain because there isn't a simple algorithm that you can follow. All you can do is look at the situation from different angles and make a decision based on the balance of the arguments presented. At an interview, the interviewers will use these ambiguities to confuse you. It is inevitable that you will end up presenting contradictory arguments, but you should always remember that this is due to the nature of the ethical dilemma rather than your own inaptitude. You must retain your confidence and use the confusion to your advantage by highlighting how this demonstrates the complexity of the problem.

10.46 A 14-year-old girl presents to you asking for a termination of pregnancy. What are the issues?

This question deals with many important concepts.

Can the girl actually have an abortion?

The first thing to do would be to confirm the pregnancy and determine how old the foetus was as, over 24 weeks, abortion is not an option. You must also take into account her competence. See Section 5.10 for full details. If the child is Fraser competent then she will be able to consent to the abortion without the need to involve her parents. If she is not Fraser competent, then you must involve her parents. You will be assessing her competence by discussing, amongst other things, the circumstances of the pregnancy with her, her understanding of contraception, of the consequences of abortion, etc. – in other words, her general maturity in relation to the circumstances.

Confidentiality

The issue of confidentiality arises if the girl is competent and refused to involve her parents. Although the issue of the abortion itself is fairly straightforward, there are other issues to consider. For example, has she been abused or raped? How old is the boyfriend? If you feel that the child is at risk then you may need to breach confidentiality (see Section 5.11) and notify the parents, or social services, or even the police in some cases. Because of the sensitive nature of the situation, you will need to remain very vigilant about the manner in which you handle the situation. Generally speaking, if you feel that a third party should be involved (for example, if you want to involve social services because she was raped), you should discuss the issue with the patient first. It is always better to come to an agreement rather than impose your own decision onto the patient (which should be your last resort). As well as saving you from breaching confidentiality, it involves the patient in the decision making process and facilitates a more successful outcome.

Holistic approach

Any girl having a child or an abortion at the age of 14 will need to be followed up in many ways. There will be:

- Physical considerations: physical impact of the abortion itself, treating any conditions linked to her sexual activity (sexually transmitted infections – STIs).
- Psychological considerations such as mental well-being prior to pregnancy, consequences of the pregnancy and of the abortion on the girl, etc.
- Social consequences including impact on her relationship with her family, with the father of the child, housing issues (e.g. if she decides to keep the child after all or if her family is rejecting her).

Education

There is a need to discuss prevention with the patient, particularly in terms of contraception and prevention of STIs.

Trust

You will only be able to achieve an optimal result if you work with the patient and you do not take a paternalistic approach. Teenagers can be volatile in their emotions and gaining the girl's trust will be crucial to the outcome. You will therefore need to ensure that you communicate with her at the right level, that you take a non-threatening attitude and that you reassure her that you are there to help her. This could be particularly difficult in situations where you have to involve third parties and breach confidentiality. But this is where Medicine becomes an art!

Important note for anti-abortion candidates

Doctors are allowed to refuse to deal with patients who request abortions or contraception if it means going against their own faith or personal principles. However, this does not exempt them from their duty of care towards the patient and, in such circumstances, they would need to refer the patient to another doctor able to deal with them in accordance with their wishes. If you belong to this category, there is no harm in mentioning it at the interview, although you would need to be very careful not to miss the point of the question, which is really to see whether you can think laterally about the issues involved. You should therefore aim to present the issues in a general sense rather than focusing too long on your own beliefs.

10.47	An elderly lady refuses to take her medication for heart failure following a recent heart attack. Not taking the medication exposes her to serious risks, including possible death. She presents to your surgery with her husband who wants you to talk some sense into her. What are the issues?

Confidentiality

The question mentions that the husband is present. You will therefore need to ensure that the lady is happy with her husband sitting in on the conversation so that you do not run the risk of breaching confidentiality by revealing information that she may wish to keep from her husband.

Beneficence vs. Autonomy

By refusing to take her medication, the lady is exposing herself to a serious risk. On one hand you need to respect her right to autonomy, i.e. the right she has to make decisions for herself. However, you also have a duty of care towards the patient and must act in her best interest. Since you cannot force her to take the medication, you must at least make sure that she has all the elements to make the most sensible decision for herself. You will achieve this by educating her about her condition, the role of the medication, the consequences of taking and not taking it, etc. This must be done in a neutral manner so that you are not seen to be coercing her into her decision.

Autonomy also means that you have to respect the patient's decision once you have tried your best. If the patient ultimately wants to die, then you will need to make sure that you accompany them as best as you can in their journey towards death.

Holistic approach

You must look beyond the obvious. Just because someone exercises their right of autonomy does not mean that you have to give up on them without trying your best. Everything has an explanation, even if you cannot understand it. There must be a reason behind her refusal to take the medication. Maybe it has unwanted side effects, maybe she is depressed, or maybe she actually wants to die.

There may also be social aspects such as not liking living at her current care home or with one of her relatives. Such a decision must have deeper rooted reasons that you must try to discover if you want to care for the patient in the best possible way.

By addressing the underlying issues, you may actually resolve her problem of non-compliance with treatment.

Competence

In some cases, the elderly lady may not be competent. You will then need to consider what she would have wanted to do if she had been competent (see Section 5.10). The relatives may help in that regard.

However, you also need to consider competence in the context of the situation. Even if you felt that she would have wanted to take the tablets, you would find it hard to enforce it upon her without committing assault if she bluntly refused. Therefore, ultimately, you will need to use your communication skills to arrive at the desired result.

| 10.48 | **What would you do if a patient came to you asking for advice about a non-conventional treatment that they had found on the internet?** |

Many candidates answer this question with "I would not want to prescribe any treatment that is not conventional." Although they are perfectly right, this does not actually address the question. The question does not ask whether you would prescribe the patient but simply states that the patient is asking for your advice. In particular, you might consider that the patient may go ahead and purchase the treatment regardless of what you think of it.

Obviously, you will not seek to recommend that he goes ahead with the new treatment, but simply mentioning this at the interview will not take you very far. There are multiple facets to this question that you must address and debate. The simplest approach is to take a thematic approach whereby you address each issue in turn, rather than a chronological approach replicating the possible consultation with the patient.

Your duty

Although the patient will make up his own mind about whether to purchase the treatment in question, you still have a duty of beneficence and non-maleficence towards the patient. The patient will have his reasons for wanting to purchase the treatment and you would need to identify what these may be. Also, you would want to make sure that the patient has all the elements in hand to make his decision. Your role in this process is therefore important. If you simply turned the patient away and patronised him, he may make the wrong decision through ignorance.

Gathering information

There are two areas where you need information: on the treatment and on the patient's reasons and hopes.

The treatment:
- What claims are being made about the treatment?
- What does it contain?
- How is it regulated? (For example, it may be non-conventional in the UK but conventional somewhere else. Any information helps).
- Ask the patient to provide you with the address of the internet site.

The patient:
- Why does the patient feel the need for this treatment?
- What problems is the current treatment causing?
- Is he intending to replace his current treatment with the new one or to take the new treatment in addition to his current one?

Once you have gathered some crucial information you will have a clearer idea about what to do.

Investigating the treatment

You may be able to find out more information about the treatment in different ways. For example, you could:
- Ask the patient to bring you one of the pills so that you can have it analysed in a lab.
- Ask some of your colleagues and pharmacists whether they have heard of the treatment.
- Contact the sellers and obtain further information.

Informing the patient

Once you have done your research, in order to act in the best interest of the patient, there are a number of messages that you will need to give him. These include:
- Addressing the concerns that the patient has expressed about his current treatment.

- A warning against information found on the internet and any claims made thereon.

- An explanation of what the product in question is and of the impact that the ingredients are likely to have on the patient.

- A warning that the product has not followed the same rigorous testing as a conventional drug would and is not approved in the UK.

- An explanation of the consequences of giving up any current conventional treatment or of taking the internet treatment in addition to any current conventional treatment (the two may interfere).

Holistic approach

The patient's needs should be fully assessed through your discussion. As well as handling the physical aspect by reviewing his current treatment if necessary, you should also address the psychological issues that the patient is facing. It may be the case that the patient's wish to move towards a non-conventional treatment is linked to the fact that they are depressed because their current conventional treatment is showing poor results. Addressing the psychological aspect may put the patient back on track. There may also be social issues. For example, the conventional treatment may stop them from enjoying their favourite hobby, or may reduce their mobility around the house. This would all need to be discussed and you may need to involve other colleagues (such as occupational therapists, physiotherapists, etc.).

Patient autonomy

Ultimately, it will be the patient's decision to carry on or terminate their current treatment. However, you must make sure that you are giving them all the information that they need to make an informed choice. While you can be assertive in presenting some of these facts, you should not be coercive.

10.49 A patient comes to see you and requests an HIV test. What do you need to think about?

The main point of asking this question is not, of course, to test your knowledge of HIV management, but to see if you can look at the situation from different angles.

There are several reasons why someone may have an HIV test. This may be a wish of their own, as in this case, or as part of other comprehensive medical investigations. The situation in which the test has been requested will obviously affect the patient's expectations of the result. In turn, this will have an impact on the way in which a positive or negative result is delivered as well and will dictate the manner in which the patient is handled prior to the test.

Although, in practice, there will be no real issue in carrying out a test, there are other matters that should cross your mind:

Why is the patient asking for a test in the first place?

Perhaps they have been exposed to a risk of catching HIV, e.g. through unprotected sex or needle sharing. If that is the case, there will be a need to educate the patient about the risks they are taking, without being patronising.

Perhaps they are simply misinformed and think they were at risk when in fact they were not (for example, some patients think you can catch HIV from a public toilet seat). In that case, the patient will need to be reassured and informed.

Timing of test

The timing of the test is very important. Some tests only detect the virus three months after the patient has been exposed to it. The fastest test has a six-week window. So the test may not cover any risk to which the patient might have been exposed in the past few weeks. That means that a negative result may not actually mean that the patient isn't infected. In such situation the patient would need to abstain from any activity which would expose him to the risk of catching the virus and come back later for further testing. (Note that you don't need to know all about specific HIV tests but having thought about the issue would be a bonus.)

How old is the patient?

If the patient is below the age of 18 and they had sex with someone much older then there may be child protection/child abuse issues, introducing a criminal element. It would be important to get from the patient an idea of how old/who their partner was.

Is the patient aware of the consequences of a positive result?

If the result is negative then the patient will undoubtedly feel relieved (though you ought to ensure that they are reminded of the risks of engaging in the behaviour which drove them to request a test in the first place). But if the results are positive, this will have a devastating effect on the patient. As a doctor, you should be prepared to handle a positive result and ensure you discuss with the patient how they would be supported and how they will cope with it.

Confidentiality

HIV is still a stigmatised disease and the patient will be undoubtedly concerned about telling others. You will need to reassure the patient that any dealings you have with them are totally confidential. You should also encourage them to gain support from those who are close to them (family, friends) so that they feel supported.

10.50	**You are a physician looking after a patient who was diagnosed with HIV a few months ago. You have encouraged him to disclose his diagnosis to his wife, which he has refused to do. What do you do?**

Beware of questions asking what you would do, since, in most cases, you cannot decide much without further information. Instead, you should concentrate your efforts on raising the issues at stake and the parameters that you would use to make decisions.

This question really is: "Should you disclose the diagnosis to his wife or not?" Ultimately, your worry will be that he is exposing his wife to the risk of HIV (e.g. through unprotected sex) or that she is already positive and is missing out on treatment.

Confidentiality and ethical dilemma

As a doctor, you have a duty of confidentiality towards your patient. This would prevent you from disclosing any information about the patient's status, including to his own GP. However, there are situations where you may be allowed to breach confidentiality; this may be possible if the patient posed a great risk to others for example (see Section 5.11).

If the wife is also one of your patients, this will complicate matters, since you will have an immediate dilemma between your duty of confidentiality towards the patient and your duty of beneficence towards his wife.

Is the wife at risk?

You should not make assumptions about the situation. Although the patient is married, he may not be having sex with his wife, and, if he is, he may be using condoms. One of your first tasks will therefore be to discuss with the patient his personal circumstances to ascertain his wife's level of exposure. On the other hand, even if he is using condoms, condoms can split and she would therefore benefit from disclosure as, should a split happen, she would require counselling and, possibly, emergency therapy to prevent HIV acquisition (PEP – Post Exposure Prophylaxis). This is all assuming that she is HIV-negative, since, if she were to be HIV-positive already, disclosure may encourage her to undergo HIV testing and allow her to benefit from medical care.

Can you make the patient change his mind?

As an empathic doctor, you will of course understand why the patient may be worried about disclosing his HIV status to his wife. Before placing the patient in a difficult position by divulging his condition to his wife, you would therefore need to have an in-depth discussion with him about his reluctance and the reasons behind it. Through counselling, possibly involving other support staff, you may be able to reassure him and guide him through the disclosure process. If ultimately he refuses outright, breaching confidentiality may be your only option.

Should you breach confidentiality?

If, given the circumstances and the information provided by the patient, you strongly suspect that his wife is at risk, then you may be entitled to breach confidentiality. Such decision would often be taken as a team and you would therefore need to confer with colleagues before going ahead. Ultimately, you will need to be confident that you can suitably justify your position in court, should you need to do so.

Before you breach confidentiality, you should encourage the patient to divulge the information to his wife by himself. In essence, you would set up a verbal contract with the patient whereby he should discuss the situation with his wife within an agreed timeframe, failing which you would undertake to divulge the information yourself. The timeframe involved would very much depend on the urgency of the situation and the risks involved.

10.51 What is your opinion on vivisection, i.e. testing on live animals?

Vivisection commonly refers to animal testing (though it literally means "cutting alive" and could apply to any living entity, including human beings). It is estimated that up to 100 million animals are used each year for research purposes, with countries having developed more or less stringent codes of conduct to regulate their use. The UK is thought to have one of the most stringent codes.

Animals are used for different purposes, including:
- Studies into development
- Studies into comportment
- Studies into evolution
- Research aiming to determine new cures and treatments
- Toxicology studies
- Cosmetics development.

Arguments in favour of animal testing

- We need to understand physiology and pathology using basic cellular studies. This can only be carried out on animals.

- We must ensure that new treatments are safe for humans. Testing on animals is essential to ensure a safe transition. Ultimately, there will always be a first human being who will take the drug in question. Not testing on animals beforehand would make that human being the first guinea pig. This would lead to even greater ethical considerations.

- Animal suffering is minimised and most do not feel anything.

- There are not many alternatives (e.g. there is only so much that a computer can simulate). Sometimes it is necessary to test in a live environment.

Arguments against animal testing

- This is depriving an animal from its normal life and is cruel. There is no reason to consider that an animal's life is less valuable than a human life.

- The animals are defenceless and cannot consent.

- It may not always lead to results that can be used (for example, parsley is a poison for parrots, morphine anaesthetises humans but excites cats, and arsenic is harmless to sheep). Recent trials at Northwick Park hospital went drastically wrong for the first few human volunteers despite the fact that tests had been carried out on animals at 500 times the dose.

- A number of tests are unnecessarily repeated. For example, if two pharmaceuticals are researching similar drugs, they will both do tests. This element of duplication might make sense from a commercial secrecy point of view, but it means that twice as many animals as necessary are being used for testing. Introducing mechanisms whereby information can be shared more efficiently would remove some of the unnecessary testing.

- There are alternatives that can be used in some cases, e.g. computer modelling or cell cultures.

The legislation

In the UK, a voluntary agreement was implemented in 1998 whereby the government would no longer issue licences to test cosmetic products or ingredients on animals. In 2009, the European Union banned the sale of products which had been tested on animals within the EU. However, the sale of products tested on animals outside of the EU remained legal, thus creating a big loophole (essentially all the legislation achieved was to stop companies carrying out the testing within the EU).

In March 2013, following 30 years of campaigning by prominent organisations, the EU introduced a total ban on the sales of products tested on animals anywhere in the world. This had an immediate impact on the behaviour of non-EU countries. In India, the drug controller issued a directive for the fast-track deletion of cosmetics animal tests. Just before the EU sales ban came in, the Japanese beauty brand Shiseido announced it would end virtually all animal testing as a direct result of the EU ban.

10.52	Do you think it is right for parents to conceive a second child to cure a disease in their first child?

Why would anyone want to do that?

There are conditions that can only be cured through the introduction of cells or organs that constitute a perfect match and for which the only realistic chance is to find a suitable relative. If no such relative is available, it is tempting to "create" one that would match.

Arguments for:

- The unique but powerful advantage is that the life of the first child may be saved by the second child.

Arguments against:

- There is no guarantee that the new child will be a suitable donor for the first child. Should this be the case, it will not only have devastating consequences for the first child but, in addition, the second child may develop a guilt complex later on in life (although it could be argued that this could easily be handled through appropriate psychotherapy if and when this occurs).

- The second child may be born with the same condition as the first child. This would have a devastating effect on the whole family.

- The primary purpose behind having the second child is effectively to produce "spare parts". This could distance the siblings and may make the second child feel that he was not born out of love but out of necessity.

- This is a slippery slope leading to possible issues of genetic selection (for example if the second child must fulfil specific criteria in order to constitute an appropriate donor).

10.53 Do you think that the government is right to impose that the NHS should only allow the MMR vaccine rather than three individual vaccines?

To answer this question you will need to be aware of the issue of MMR vaccination (see Section 5.2).

In your discussion you should consider the following facts:

- The fact that the studies showing a link to autism have pretty much been disproved.

- The combined vaccine is safer and more effective as children are not put at risk of catching the diseases while they are waiting for full immunisation.

- The role of the NHS is to offer what is believed to be the best solution to a particular health issue taking into account cost considerations. In this case, patients are actually offered a choice in that they can still get the three vaccines separately albeit on a private basis (i.e. they have to pay for them out of their own pocket). This is a good compromise to ensure that patients can exercise their choice, while ensuring that the nation provides the solution of choice free of charge.

10.54	**You are a junior doctor and, just before the morning ward round, you notice that your consultant smells of alcohol. What do you do?**

This question is becoming increasingly frequent as it enables interviewers to test your flexibility in dealing with a difficult and sensitive issue, your empathy, your team playing abilities and also your integrity. To answer this question successfully, you must consider a number of issues:

Patient safety

As a doctor, patient safety will always be your first priority (except where your own safety is compromised in which case it will come first).

Because your consultant is drunk, you will need to ensure that he is not dealing with patients (dangerous enough for a medic, even more dangerous for a surgeon) and that he leaves the ward. Since you are a junior, it is easier said than done, but in reality you will have other people around you to help: for example a senior nurse, another trainee doctor or even another consultant. This will need to be handled discreetly and sensitively so as not to alert patients and not to embarrass the consultant in question in front of others.

Also in the interest of patient safety, you will need to ensure that the patients the consultant has already seen, or for whom he has made decisions, are reviewed by someone else. Once the consultant has been removed from the clinical area, you will need to ensure that patient care is appropriately covered and that the team can cope with the absence of the consultant. You will need to involve other doctors and managers to ensure appropriate cover.

As an aside you will also need to look after your colleague's safety by ensuring that he is okay and by booking a taxi to send him home so that he does not take the gamble of driving back, or by organising a room where he can sleep it off.

Reporting the matter

Whatever the reasons behind the consultant's behaviour, the fact that he turned up at work drunk (when most people would have called in sick) shows a serious lack of judgement that could have a devastating impact on patients. It will therefore be a matter for someone of higher authority to deal with.

You would benefit greatly by reading the GMC's *Good Medical Practice,* which can be accessed online via www.gmc-uk.org, as it contains information that could prove valuable at an interview. Section 23 is clear that if you believe that a doctor is placing patients at risk you have a duty to report your concerns with someone in authority.[3] There will most likely be guidelines within your Trust, in which case you should follow them, but if there are not then you should adopt the most logical route. In either case, your next step will most likely be to discuss the situation with another consultant or the clinical director (i.e. the head of your department) and let them handle the situation.

Supporting the team and your colleague

The team will inevitably suffer the consequences of the situation. For example, the consultant may be asked to take some time off, to go on lighter duties, etc. and you will need to make sure that you have a flexible attitude that enables the team to function well despite the problem. Whenever possible, you should also offer your personal support to your colleague in your own way.

Communicating

Throughout the situation, you will need to demonstrate sensitivity and care not to disrupt the team more than necessary. You should be understanding towards the consultant rather than critical and understand that there may be real issues and personal drama behind the situation. This means that you should also aim to minimise his embarrassment by not spreading gossip and only discussing the matter with relevant people.

What if it is the first time?

There is no proof that this is a first incident. It may have happened in previous jobs (look at Dr Shipman – see Section 5.1). It may be happening in private and you might simply have witnessed the first incident at work, but it still remains that, without your intervention, patients may have suffered. The approach is therefore the same, first time or not.

---

[3] http://www.gmc-uk.org/guidance/good_medical_practice/respond_to_risks.asp

What if he had a "good" reason to be drunk? What if he pleads with you not to say anything?

There may be several reasons for someone to turn up drunk at work. The consultant may have a personal problem (his wife left him, his mother died, etc.) or maybe he simply drank too much at a party. If there are miti- gating circumstances, then they will be taken into account by the senior person who handles the matter. But you should not attempt to cover up something as serious as this on the basis that you feel sorry for the con- sultant. If there is a problem, you can be understanding and empathic but it is not really up to you to resolve it. It is an issue that he will need to deal with personally with the help of the department; hence why a senior col- league should be involved.

If the consultant has a real alcohol problem, you will not do him any fa- vours by covering up for him. In fact, if something happened later which could have been prevented if you had said something earlier, then you would find yourself in front of the GMC for negligence/breach of duty.

What if, despite reporting the matter, nothing happens and he does it again?

First, do not jump to conclusions. Although it may not seem like it, your seniors are probably handling the matter but they can't always keep an eye on the consultant. If the problem recurs, talk to them again and see what they say. If at any stage you feel uncomfortable with the situation, you can always choose to escalate the matter but you must do so care- fully. Before escalating further (for example to the medical director or the chief executive), you may find a way to seek advice from other colleagues or even from special helplines for doctors, which many institutions run. Your final resort will be the relevant Royal College and the GMC.

What if he is your best friend?

Whether he is your best friend or not does not change anything about the gravity of the situation. The only difference it will make is in the communi- cation skills that you will use. If the consultant is your best friend, you may be more inclined to spend a longer period of time talking to him about the consequences of his actions at the beginning. But your friend will also need to accept responsibility and understand the position in which you find yourself.

10.55 What would you do if a colleague asked you to prescribe them some antidepressants?

This question is interesting and misinterpreted by many candidates. Too often, candidates rush into answering that they would not prescribe for a colleague because it is illegal. Not only is this not entirely correct, it also fails to address the multiple facets of the question. The question is not just asking about prescription but specifically mentions antidepressants. Ask yourself why he may be requesting these drugs and you will open up a whole new line of thought.

Prescribing for friends and family

Strictly speaking it is not illegal for doctors to prescribe for friends and family (the GMC's guidance is in fact that "Wherever possible you must avoid prescribing for yourself or anyone with whom you have a close personal relationship"[4]); although of course such practice is not best practice. There are several reasons for this including:

- It is open to abuse.
- There is no centralised approach to the care of the person being prescribed in the way that there would be if that person went to their GP instead.

Note that only a few doctors are allowed to prescribe controlled drugs such as antidepressants. This includes GPs and psychiatrists. Therefore even if you were tempted to write a prescription, you would not be able to.

Your colleague's need

You would need to establish why your colleague needs the antidepressants and why he is not going to his GP to obtain a prescription. Reasons might include:

- He may not have the time to go to his GP, in which case what you should really do is to ensure that he finds the time to do so: for example by swapping shifts or by encouraging him to discuss the matter with a senior colleague.

---

[4] http://www.gmc-uk.org/guidance/ethical_guidance/14318.asp

- He may be retailing the drugs to addicts, in which case he would not be honest with you and you certainly would not want to be part of it.
- He may be depressed but wants to keep it outside the normal system because he is worried that it may affect his job. In this case, you would need to reassure him about the confidentiality of the GP service and encourage him to seek proper help. You would also want to explain to him that it is better to address the problem at an early stage than let it develop into an even bigger problem.

Whatever the situation, he really needs to see a GP and maybe seek specialist help, but you are not the best person to address the issue. He will need to be properly assessed and prescribed by relevant specialists rather than prescribed in 2 minutes in the corridor by you without any appropriate background.

Fitness to practise and patient safety

There is a possibility that his depression is affecting his ability to function normally at work and you will need to address this with him too. In particular, rather than report this straight away to senior colleagues, you may want to encourage your colleague to see a senior colleague himself and discuss the matter with them so that they can derive ways of helping him out.

If you feel that your colleague presents a danger to patients and does not want to address the situation then you may have no option but to discuss the matter yourself with senior colleagues.

Supporting your colleague and the team

If your colleague is going through a difficult time, you should show support. This could be either at a personal level by offering your time to discuss his problems or by helping the team and him to deal with any consequences (e.g. being flexible and taking on more work for a while, etc.). Empathy and teamwork are two important skills to demonstrate.

10.56 What would you do if you caught a colleague looking at child pornography on a computer at work?

The situation here is different from the scenario of the drunk consultant in two respects:

- The situation does not present an <u>immediate</u> danger to patients through his actions, although it would be a valid argument to say that the doctor presents a danger to children in general anyway.

- His activities are illegal.

The approach

Your approach will consist of the following steps:

- Take note of the date and time when you have seen the colleague use the computer. This will be needed for the hospital to prove the case against the colleague.

- Discuss the situation with a colleague you trust if you need support and report the matter to a senior colleague. They, in turn, should notify management and the police once they are satisfied that there are reasonable grounds to do so.

- Support the team. Reporting the colleague will certainly lead to some form of disciplinary action and probable dismissal. The team will need to pull together to cope with the change.

- If you feel that action is slow (for example the incident recurs despite repeated complaints) then you should follow up, and escalate further if nothing is being done.

- If you do not know what to do or are worried about the consequences for you, you can seek advice from relevant helplines.

What if the pornography is adult pornography?

If the pornography is not child pornography then the matter is entirely different as it would not be illegal. Although he may be breaching hospital policy (which is a matter for the hospital to sort out), your main concern would really be whether his actions are actually compromising patient safety.

Your first step would probably be to have a chat with your colleague. He would need to realise that he is endangering his reputation and his career if he got caught. If you don't know him then you will need to make a decision as to whether you need to report him or not.

Issues to consider would include:

- Is there a policy in place in the Trust and, particularly, would you be in trouble if you did not report the matter?

- Is the doctor in question actually compromising patient care? After all, although looking at pornography and abusing NHS resources may not be acceptable in the workplace, he is not committing an illegal act. If, however, the doctor were compromising the care of his patients at any time or acting against the interest of the team (for example by spending too much time on the computer), then you would have strong grounds to report the matter to a senior colleague.

Ultimately, it will be left to your judgement depending on the nature of the situation.

10.57   Under what circumstances would it be acceptable to lie?

You will need to handle this question carefully to get the right message across and, more importantly, you will need to separate what one would consider acceptable in "normal life" and what one would consider acceptable as a doctor.

Normal life

In normal life, people often lie to protect themselves (e.g. telling a teacher that you did not do an assignment because of some obscure reason); to protect others' feelings ("No, your bum does not look big in this dress", "The Joneses told me they had a really nice time when they came to our party"); or to gain a personal advantage (e.g. financial – "Yes this is the right car for you").

The first two lies are often "white lies" and are usually harmless, though getting found out may affect the trust that someone has in someone else. The third one is deception, which may have more serious consequences (e.g. people being offered products they don't need including credit, insurance, etc.). It is a given that most people lie occasionally, often just to spare embarrassment, and that it is therefore an accepted part of living within a society. This does not mean that it should be acceptable (I will let you make up your own mind on that based on your own value system), but simply that it is accepted by most.

As a doctor

When you deal with patients, the consequences of a lie, even small, could be serious. Most of the trust that patients have in you as their doctor relies on the fact that they assume you will not be lying to them; therefore telling a lie to a patient could have devastating consequences.

Lying to a patient (for example by reassuring them that a procedure is safe, when in fact it presents risks, even if minimal) alters the choices they make about their own healthcare.

Some doctors have been known to lie within their research results, for example by deliberately falsifying results or omitting to divulge inconvenient results. Such lies could lead to very serious results such as drugs being used when they are in fact unsafe and, generally speaking, decisions being made on the wrong basis.

One situation where it may be "acceptable" to lie is when telling the truth may breach the confidentiality of the patient. For example, a relative may ask you to divulge information about diagnosis, prognosis, treatment options, etc. In most cases, you should really state that you are not at liberty to discuss the matter without the consent of the patient and leave it at that. However, in some cases (e.g. if there is a risk the relatives might become aggressive), it may be easier to say that you simply don't have the information. Note, however, that in such situations the lie is not meant to mislead the other person (e.g. by giving a different diagnosis to the real one) but is simply a white lie to avoid a confrontation and avoid revealing information.

Lying vs. withholding information

In Medicine, outright lies (i.e. deliberately giving false information to a direct question being posed) would always be considered unacceptable. If a patient that you know has cancer asks "Do I have cancer", you would be required to tell the truth.

There is, however, a grey area with regard to withholding information, particularly when the divulging of the information might do the patient more harm than good. For example, a patient who threatens to commit suicide should they be diagnosed with a particular illness would need careful handling. On one hand, they would need to be made aware of their diagnosis because it would be in their best interest to receive treatment; on the other hand, you would want to save them from themselves. As such, the diagnosis might be delayed for a while until the right circumstances are found.

Similarly, there may be some very elderly people who may find it hard to cope with a particular diagnosis and from whom the information may best be withheld, particularly if there is no chance of getting appropriate treatment.

However, such decision (essentially a lie by omission) would only be taken if doctors felt that disclosing the information would do more harm than good. Such instances would be rare. And, if the patient were to ask a direct question, you would most likely need to be truthful.

10.58 What can cause a doctor-patient relationship to deteriorate?

In this question, there are two protagonists: a patient and a doctor. You should therefore consider both sides:

From the patient's point of view

- The doctor is rude and patronising
- The doctor is not a good listener
- The doctor is not explaining the issues well
- The doctor is trying to rush the patient into making decisions
- The doctor is pushing the patient to make a decision that is not acceptable
- The doctor is not offering the options that the patient wants (e.g. a patient requesting antibiotics for a viral illness)
- The doctor has lied

From the doctor's point of view

- The patient is rude or aggressive
- The patient is racist
- The patient is constantly changing his mind
- The patient is lying
- The patient is constantly not adhering to the recommended treatment
- The patient is constantly querying or contradicting what the doctor says

Note that the threshold at which a patient can decide that the relationship has deteriorated is inevitably lower than for a doctor to make that same decision.

For example, if a doctor was found to have lied to a patient, there would be an immediate loss of trust and the patient could reasonably ask to be treated by a different doctor. However, it is not uncommon for patients to lie to doctors (for example, about what they eat, how much they smoke, how much exercise they do, whether they take their medication, etc.). A doctor would need to work with it before deciding that they can no longer treat that patient.

10.59 What are the causes of obesity and how can we stop the obesity crisis?

Most cases of obesity are caused by overeating and lack of exercise. Essentially, the surplus energy that is absorbed as food is not burnt off through exercise and will be turned into fat.

Poor diet

Obesity usually develops gradually from poor diet and lifestyle choices. Unhealthy food choices include:

- Processed or fast food high in fat
- Not eating fruit, vegetables and unrefined carbohydrates (e.g. wholemeal bread and brown rice)
- Drinking too much alcohol – alcohol contains a lot of calories, and heavy drinkers are often overweight
- Eating out a lot – you may have a starter or dessert in a restaurant, and the food can be higher in fat and sugar
- Eating larger portions than you need – you may be encouraged to eat too much if your friends or relatives are also eating large portions
- Comfort eating – if you feel depressed or have low self-esteem you may comfort eat to make yourself feel better.

Unhealthy eating habits tend to run in families, as you learn bad eating habits from your parents.

Lack of physical activity

Lack of physical activity is another important factor related to obesity. Many people have jobs that involve sitting at a desk most of the day. They also rely on their cars rather than walking, or cycling. When they relax, people tend to watch TV, browse the internet or play computer games, and rarely take regular exercise. If you are not active enough, you do not use the energy provided by the food you eat, and the extra calories are stored as fat instead. The Department of Health recommends adults do at least 2 hours and 30 minutes of moderate-intensity aerobic activity (i.e. cycling or fast walking) every week. However, if you are obese and trying to lose weight, you may need to do more exercise – in some cases up to 5 hours may be recommended.

Genetics

Some people claim there is no point in losing weight because "it runs in my family" or "it is in my genes". While there are some rare genetic conditions that can cause obesity, such as Prader-Willi syndrome, there is no reason why most people cannot lose weight. It may be true that certain genetic traits inherited from your parents, such as taking longer to burn up calories (having a slow metabolism) or having a large appetite, can make losing weight more difficult. But it certainly does not make it impossible. Many cases where obesity runs in families may be due to environmental factors such as poor eating habits learned during childhood.

Medical reasons

Medical conditions that can cause weight gain include:

- Cushing's syndrome (a rare disorder that causes over-production of steroid hormones)
- An underactive thyroid gland (hypothyroidism), when your thyroid gland does not produce enough thyroid hormone.

Certain medicines, including some corticosteroids and antidepressants, can also contribute to weight gain. Weight gain can also be a side effect of taking the combined contraceptive pill, and from quitting smoking.

How to stop the obesity crisis

The short answer is to get people to eat less, more healthily and take more exercise. Most of that can be done through:

- Education (via schools, youth clubs, GPs, etc.)
- Raising awareness through advertising (e.g. TV)
- Better labelling of food for high fat content
- Taxation (the government is also discussing the possibility of taxing certain food items (e.g. fizzy drinks) more heavily, though such topics are always controversial because any attempt to tax unhealthy food items is often labelled a "tax on the poor").

One major issue is that the behaviours of children tend to be copied from their parents and, therefore, unless the parents are also altering their attitude towards eating and exercise, the fight will be hard.

10.60	**What are the arguments for and against the decriminalisation of drugs such as cocaine?**

Arguments against

1. Legalisation would result in significant increases in drug use. We know that currently legal drugs, such as alcohol and tobacco, are widely consumed and associated with an extensive economic burden to society – including hospital admissions, alcoholism treatment programmes and public nuisance. So why create an environment where this may also come to pass for currently illegal drugs?

2. The moral argument against legalisation suggests the use of illegal drugs is amoral, antisocial and otherwise not acceptable in today's society. The concern is that legalisation would "send the wrong message".

3. Recent research suggests that the use of drugs is on the decline, which suggests either that prevention is working or that drugs are simply going out of fashion.

Arguments for

1. The market for drugs is demand-led and millions of people demand illegal drugs. Making the production, supply and use of some drugs illegal creates a vacuum into which organised crime moves. The profits are worth billions of pounds. Legalisation forces organised crime from the drugs trade, starves them of income and enables society to regulate and control the market (i.e. prescription, licensing, laws on sales to minors, advertising regulations, etc.).

2. To fund a habit made expensive by criminalisation, some dependent users resort to stealing to raise funds (accounting for 50% of UK property crime – estimated at £2 billion a year). Most of the violence associated with illegal drug dealing is caused by its illegality. Legalisation would enable us to regulate the market, determine a much lower price and remove users' needs to raise funds through crime. Our legal system would be freed up and our prison population dramatically reduced, saving billions. Because of the low price, cigarette smokers do not have to steal to support their habits. There is also no violence associated with the legal tobacco market.

3. Decriminalising drugs would move the problem away from police and the criminal justice system and concentrate responses within health. In addition the cost of dealing with the consequences of drugs could be met through taxation of drugs (in the same way that cigarettes are taxed).

4. Legalisation would help to disseminate open, honest and truthful information to users and non-users to help them to make decisions about whether and how to use. We could begin research again on presently illicit drugs to discover all their uses and effects – both positive and negative.

5. Prohibition has led to the stigmatisation and marginalisation of drug users. Countries that operate ultra-prohibitionist policies have very high rates of HIV infection amongst injecting users. Hepatitis C rates amongst users in the UK are increasing substantially. In the UK in the 1980s, clean needles for injecting users and safer sex education for young people were made available in response to fears of HIV. Harm reduction policies are in direct opposition to prohibitionist laws.

6. Prohibition hides the need to address the social and economic factors that lead people to use drugs. Most illegal and legal drug use is recreational. Poverty and despair are at the root of most problematic drug use and it is only by addressing these underlying causes that we can hope to significantly decrease the number of problematic users. Criminalising drugs is not addressing the underlying issues.

10.61 Do you think doctors should ever go on strike?

Arguments for

1. If an employer (such as a hospital trust) knew that doctors could not strike, this may lead to abuse such as forcing doctors to work longer hours than they are contracted to. Similarly the government could take liberties such as not increasing salaries, increasing pension contributions or imposing other reforms without fearing any consequences.

2. Not all doctors provide services that would suffer greatly if they went on strike. For example, closing a clinic for one day may simply delay the care of patients and cause an inconvenience to patients (which is after all the point of a strike) but won't cause a major disaster. Closing A&E for a day may cause more issues, however.

3. Doctors should be treated as equal to other civil servants, who are allowed to strike.

4. Hospital bosses know that, at the end of the day, strike or no strike, the same patients will need to be seen. If doctors go on strike, all patients who have been cancelled will simply be rebooked onto a different day, making those days busier and more intense. So essentially doctors will simply have to work harder on different days to make up for the lack of work on strike day.

Arguments against

1. Some patients may be severely affected (and even die) as a result of a strike. That would be the case for any emergency services. As a result, any strike can only be confined to non-emergency services.

2. Doctors are paid well and the public knows it. A strike could lead the general public to lose confidence in a profession which, though already well off, cannot share the burden of austerity with everyone else.

Important note:

In 2012, the British Medical Association organised a strike for doctors to complain about a sudden large increase in pension contributions. The public reacted with contempt to the strike because it came at a time of austerity when much less well off people had to accept pay cuts, benefit cuts and other austerity measures.

In addition, many doctors were aware that striking would only present them in a bad light to the hospital bosses and may affect their own career development. They were also acutely aware that striking would only place a greater burden on them on other days.

Finally, striking means that you don't get paid.

Consequently the strike was poorly followed.

11 Wacky questions!

In several medical schools (e.g. Hull York), you may be asked questions that are designed to test your creativity, innovation and flexibility. These questions may be regarded as "weird" by many applicants but are simply designed to see how imaginative and flexible you can be in your thinking process.

The main thing you need to remember when you are faced with such a question is that there is no right or wrong answer. In fact, the more resourceful and inventive you are, the better. In other words, wacky questions call for wacky answers!

For these questions, the main emphasis is on finding ideas, i.e. brainstorming. There is little technique to learn in terms of structuring your answers. Because of this, under each question we have listed points that were made at interviews by successful candidates and added some of our own.

Feel free to add your own to the list. For each point, give a few lines of explanation so that the interviewers understand not only what you are trying to say but also your justification.

11.1 Imagine a world in 200 years where doctors no longer exist. In what ways do you think they could be replaced?

1. Nowadays, many patients self-diagnose via the internet. Wikipedia + a good search engine could replace many doctors when it comes to diagnosing people.

2. As surgery becomes more streamlined and uses more robots, perhaps we can envisage a world where there will be no need for human intervention in surgery; and if we need human intervention, this could be performed by well-trained barbers, as it was 300 years ago. We are going full circle.

3. Currently it takes time to do blood tests as they have to be sent to a lab. The same goes for X-rays and other imaging devices. Given the pace at which smartphones are developing, it is not impossible that we will just be able to place blood or urine on a pad/chip that can be analysed by our phones, with the results being run by a central online computer.

4. Since we have managed to decode the human genome, we may be able to computerise the data onto one main computer to predict what diseases we may get in future and prevent their occurrence using information or therapies commonly available.

5. In 200 years' time we will all be living until we are 200 years old and so we will all have plenty of time to study several degrees. Everyone will basically have studied Medicine at some stage in their lifetime (that would only take 10-15 years out of the 200). Doctors would no longer exist because we would all be medically qualified, self-treating and self-medicating.

6. The way things are going in the world, it's not just doctors who will no longer exist. No one else will either!

7. Every human will have microchips implanted in their bodies, and capsules floating in the blood, which will diagnose and medicate accordingly.

11.2 You are holding a party with a medical theme. How would you make it memorable?

1. Play nurses and doctors but with reversed roles, i.e. doctors wearing nurses' uniforms and vice versa.

2. Serve hospital food!

3. Use only medical implements, e.g. Petri dishes for plates, scalpels for knives, and bedpans for the chocolate mousse!

4. Shape the food as body parts, e.g. cakes in the shape of brains, etc. (beware of the examples you give for this one!) and serve the drinks in syringes.

5. Give everyone laughing gas (normally used for anaesthetic purposes so clearly that one poses some serious ethical problems).

11.3 Describe as many uses as you can for a mobile phone charger

If you keep the plug attached

- Charging mobile phones!

- Sling (especially if the plug is heavy)

- Plug-in air freshener giving an absolutely neutral smell

- Plug protector for babies

- Fishing implement

If you leave the plug aside

In that case, all you get is the cord and you can use it to replace anything that can be achieved with a piece of string, for example:

- Tourniquet

- Shoe laces

- Bracelet

- Drive belt

- Measurement unit

- Making scoobies

- Plant ties

11.4 Imagine you had six months with enough money and nothing you had to do. Tell us the most imaginative (and non-medical) way in which you would spend your time

With this question you have to be a little careful. This was asked at Hull York Medical School in the category "Innovation and Imagination" but if you get asked that type of question in any other medical school you will need to make sure you are clear about the wording.

The reason for our warning is that this could be easily answered in a similar way to "Tell us about your hobbies" (see Q.9.14). However, here the question is specifically asking about the "most imaginative way", allowing you to exercise a bit more artistic licence.

Having said that you could also link your answer to some of your current interests.

Here are a few examples of answers that would work (and have worked):

- Someone who enjoyed drawing, painting and teaching said they would really like to set up an arts class for deprived people in their area. This would keep them out of trouble, would enable them to express their emotions through an artistic medium and would also teach them valuable skills.

- Someone with a passion for astronomy (not astrology!) said that they would want to go fund-raising to buy a place on the Virgin galactic flight. He then went on to describe the various ways in which he could raise the $200,000 required.

- Someone with an interest in cooking and travel described how she would write a book on a particular type of cookery, including sourcing rare ingredients in the UK.

- Someone discussed how they had always wanted to own a restaurant in Italy and that they would use the 6 months to try their idea out.

You could use your own examples to showcase some of your own personal skills (e.g. your organisational skills, your ability to work with others, etc.).

11.5 If you were shipwrecked on a desert island with all your physical needs – such as food and water – taken care of, what three items would you like to take with you?

Three items is not actually that much when you consider that you need some basics and something to entertain yourself too.

There are items that there is no point in taking, such as toothpaste (if you are destined to stay on that island, what will you do once your tube has run out?) or a chainsaw (even if you take some petrol with you it won't last long – a hacksaw may be more useful).

Items could include:

- Practical items such as a saw (you don't need a hammer, you can use coconuts or stones for that, whereas making a saw is a bit more problematic), or a pair of pliers.

- Useful books such as a survival manual (how to fish, how to hunt, etc.) or a religious book if you are religious, or a particularly inspiring collection of poems or sayings which may help you keep your motivation level up. Try to avoid novels or any single-use item.

- Comfort items, e.g. a blanket.

Ideally you will offer a mix of practical and comfort items so that you appear clued up and human at the same time. Explain why you would choose or not choose specific items so that they can follow your logic.

11.6	**Do you think that sending a man to the moon was money well spent?**

This question is disarming at first because it does not seem terribly relevant to Medicine. However, it is quite explicitly about how to allocate money from a national budget (sound familiar?).

Many candidates rush into answering the question by saying that the trip to the moon did not achieve much and that the money could have been better spent on the health service. Although this is a good argument in itself, it is a little simplistic for this type of interview and there are many more aspects to consider. For example:

- When you go shopping for food or for clothes, do you always buy the cheapest items in order to give the money that you saved to your favourite charity or to the NHS?

- Do you refrain from offering presents to friends and family because that money is really a luxury and could be better utilised for the good of society?

In most cases, the answer would be, of course, "no". So, along the same lines, why should a government spend all its money on the health service? We spend money on putting flowers on roundabouts. Is this a luxury or a need? One could argue that it has an important psychological impact on the population.

This question is all about what society is seeking to achieve and how the right balance can be maintained between the "useful" and the "luxuries".

Here are a few arguments that should help you in your discussion:

- Space exploration is an important element in building a future for the human race. It has to start somewhere and the technology developed to place a man on the moon has been a very successful start.

- The successful moon missions have considerably boosted the morale of the nations involved. It can easily be argued that the general well-being of a population and a healthy degree of patriotism are important factors too and that a nation should be able to afford such luxuries.

347

- Space exploration may lead to scientific discoveries that could actually help the advancement of Medicine. This may not be immediately apparent but the rewards may be reaped at a later stage.

- The space race encouraged competition between nations and ensured a fast track technological advancement. However, it could also be argued that such a level of competition at times proved to be unhealthy, particularly during the cold war.

- Of course, it could be argued that the money could be better spent on more worthy causes, such as a better health system. On the other hand, it could be argued that, rather than investing money into the health system, one should aim to make it more efficient with its current budget. Injecting more money into healthcare does not necessarily lead to better results. It might even lead to greater inefficiencies and complacency.

- Resources could have been used to tackle poverty. There is no arguing with this, though it raises the same question about the efficiency of current funding and whether throwing more money at it would actually achieve better results.

- If we take the stance that every luxury should be sacrificed in favour of a state-of-the-art health system, people would be well looked after but would be miserable and depressed!

12 Action & Power Words

Here is a list of over 500 power words that you can use to increase the strength of your answers. These can be used not only in formal interview questions but also in role play and group discussions.

Abbreviated	Abolished	Abridged	Absolved
Absorbed	Accelerated	Acclimated	Accompanied
Achieved	Acquired	Acted	Activated
Actuated	Adapted	Added	Addressed
Adhered	Adjusted	Administered	Admitted
Adopted	Advanced	Advertised	Advised
Advocated	Affected	Aided	Aired
Allocated	Altered	Amended	Amplified
Analysed	Answered	Anticipated	Applied
Appointed	Appraised	Approached	Approved
Arbitrated	Arranged	Articulated	Ascertained
Asked	Assembled	Assessed	Assigned
Assisted	Assumed	Attained	Attracted
Audited	Augmented	Authored	Authorised
Awarded	Balanced	Began	Benchmarked
Benefited	Bid	Billed	Blocked
Boosted	Borrowed	Bought	Branded
Bridged	Broadened	Brought	Budgeted
Built	Calculated	Canvassed	Captured
Cared	Cast	Catalogued	Categorised
Centralised	Chaired	Challenged	Changed
Channelled	Charged	Charted	Checked
Circulated	Clarified	Classified	Cleared
Closed	Coached	Co-authored	Collaborated
Collected	Combined	Commissioned	Committed
Communicated	Compared	Compiled	Completed
Complied	Composed	Computed	Conceived
Conceptualised	Condensed	Conducted	Conserved

Consolidated	Constructed	Consulted	Contacted
Contributed	Controlled	Converted	Conveyed
Convinced	Coordinated	Copyrighted	Corrected
Corresponded	Counselled	Created	Critiqued
Cultivated	Customised	Cut	Dealt
Debated	Debugged	Decentralised	Decreased
Deferred	Defined	Delegated	Delivered
Demonstrated	Depreciated	Described	Designated
Designed	Detected	Determined	Developed
Devised	Diagnosed	Directed	Discovered
Dispatched	Dissembled	Distinguished	Distributed
Diversified	Divested	Documented	Doubled
Drove	Earned	Eased	Edited
Educated	Effected	Elicited	Eliminated
Emphasised	Empowered	Enabled	Encouraged
Endorsed	Enforced	Engaged	Engineered
Enhanced	Enlarged	Enlisted	Enriched
Ensured	Escalated	Established	Estimated
Evaluated	Examined	Exceeded	Exchanged
Executed	Exempted	Expanded	Expedited
Experienced	Explained	Explored	Exposed
Extended	Extracted	Fabricated	Facilitated
Fashioned	Fielded	Financed	Fired
Flagged	Focused	Forecasted	Formalised
Formatted	Formed	Formulated	Fortified
Founded	Fulfilled	Furnished	Furthered
Gained	Gathered	Gauged	Generated
Governed	Graded	Granted	Greeted
Grouped	Guided	Handled	Headed
Helped	Hired	Hosted	Identified
Ignited	Illuminated	Illustrated	Impacted
Implemented	Improved	Improvised	Inaugurated
Incorporated	Increased	Incurred	Individualised
Indoctrinated	Induced	Influenced	Initiated
Innovated	Inquired	Inspected	Inspired
Installed	Instigated	Instilled	Instituted
Instructed	Insured	Integrated	Interacted
Interpreted	Intervened	Interviewed	Introduced

Invented	Inventoried	Invested	Investigated
Invited	Involved	Isolated	Issued
Joined	Judged	Justified	Kept
Launched	Lectured	Led	Lightened
Liquidated	Litigated	Lobbied	Localised
Located	Logged	Maintained	Managed
Manufactured	Mapped	Marketed	Maximised
Measured	Mediated	Mentored	Merchandised
Merged	Minimised	Modelled	Moderated
Modernised	Modified	Monitored	Motivated
Moved	Multiplied	Named	Narrated
Navigated	Negotiated	Netted	Noticed
Nourished	Nursed	Nurtured	Observed
Obtained	Offered	Opened	Operated
Orchestrated	Ordered	Organised	Oriented
Originated	Overhauled	Oversaw	Participated
Patented	Patterned	Performed	Persuaded
Phased	Photographed	Pinpointed	Pioneered
Placed	Planned	Polled	Posted
Prepared	Presented	Preserved	Presided
Prevented	Processed	Procured	Produced
Proficient	Profiled	Programmed	Projected
Promoted	Prompted	Proposed	Prospected
Proved	Provided	Publicised	Published
Purchased	Pursued	Qualified	Quantified
Quoted	Raised	Ranked	Rated
Received	Recognised	Recommended	Reconciled
Recorded	Recovered	Recruited	Rectified
Redesigned	Reduced	Referred	Refined
Regained	Registered	Regulated	Rehabilitated
Reinforced	Reinstated	Rejected	Remedied
Remodelled	Renegotiated	Reorganised	Repaired
Replaced	Reported	Represented	Rescued
Researched	Resolved	Responded	Restored
Restructured	Resulted	Retained	Retrieved
Revamped	Revealed	Reversed	Reviewed
Revised	Revitalised	Rewarded	Safeguarded
Salvaged	Saved	Scheduled	Screened

Secured	Segmented	Selected	Separated
Served	Serviced	Settled	Shaped
Shortened	Shrank	Signed	Simplified
Simulated	Sold	Solicited	Solved
Spearheaded	Specialised	Specified	Speculated
Spoke	Spread	Stabilised	Staffed
Staged	Standardised	Steered	Stimulated
Strategised	Streamlined	Strengthened	Stressed
Structured	Studied	Submitted	Substantiated
Substituted	Suggested	Superseded	Supervised
Supplied	Supported	Surpassed	Surveyed
Synchronised	Systematised	Tabulated	Tailored
Targeted	Taught	Tested	Tightened
Took	Traced	Tracked	Traded
Trained	Transacted	Transcribed	Transferred
Transformed	Translated	Transmitted	Transported
Treated	Tripled	Troubleshot	Tutored
Uncovered	Underlined	Undertook	Unearthed
Unified	United	Updated	Upgraded
Urged	Used	Utilised	Validated
Valued	Verbalised	Verified	Viewed
Visited	Visualised	Voiced	Volunteered
Weathered	Weighed	Welcomed	Widened
Withstood	Witnessed	Won	Worked
Wrote	Yielded		

MMI

PRACTICAL

STATIONS

13 Written task/ Questionnaire

In some cases, the interviewers feel that it is more productive to avoid using a face-to-face interview format to ask some of the more mundane questions and prefer to ask candidates to answer those in writing.

Usually candidates are given 30 minutes or so to answer 2 or 3 questions of the type:

- Why do you want to be a doctor?
- Why this medical school?
- What qualities do you possess that will make you a good doctor?

The questions asked are often the most predictable ones (i.e. you will no doubt have thought about them before) and therefore finding the appropriate content should not be a challenge.

However, there are two issues you need to be aware of:

1. A written answer will need to be more formal than a verbal answer, i.e. you may need to use slightly different words and sometimes grammar. So, for example, if your oral answer contained a sentence such as "After school I regularly teach pupils from a local school how to read and write – they are not always easy to manage, but I really enjoy it", your written answer should read "After school I regularly teach pupils from a local school how to read and write. Although they are not always easy to manage, I really enjoy it."

2. It is possible that your handwriting may be checked for legibility (they certainly check when it comes to application forms, which doctors complete for their own job applications. So make sure you take your time to write a neat form. If you have spare paper available, use it to draw a quick plan for your answer before writing on the proper form.

14 Discussion around a newspaper article

Increasingly, newspaper articles or online articles are used to test candidates' ability to debate important issues and formulate arguments. The newspaper articles usually relate to ethical dilemmas and court cases recently (last 12-18 months) reported on by the press.

Examples of cases or issues that have come up at interviews included the following:

1. **The parents of a severely disabled teenage girl who wanted their daughter to have her womb and ovaries removed to stop her having her periods.**

   In this case the debate was about the rights of the child vs. the rights and comfort of the parents. It was also about whether, by making it easier for the parents to look after their child, this would in fact benefit the child (despite the fact she would be forced to have an operation without being able to give consent herself).

2. **Smokers and obese patients being taken off the NHS waiting lists because other patients who did not smoke and had a normal weight were deemed to be more suitable candidates.**

   This led to discussion on the basic ethical principles of beneficence, maleficence and justice (see Section 5.8), as well as the issues of rationing, the need for patients to take charge of their own well-being, and the role of doctors and the state in prevention and education.

3. **The parents of a child who needed a transplant but with the only donor possible being a sibling. The parents had therefore had a second child specifically with the aim of acting as a donor for the first child.**

   The discussions revolved around the morality of conceiving the second child or the sole purpose of saving the first one. Candidates were also asked how they felt the parents would feel about their second child, how the second child would feel if he found out the truth (Understanding? Complex of superiority? Wanting to make the first child grateful for saving his life? etc.), and how the first child would feel about the second child when he was older (Grateful? Inferior? Shameful? etc.).

4. **A daughter who had taken her father to die in a clinic in Switzerland and had been condemned to a 12-month suspended jail sentence.**

    The debate revolved around the pros and cons of euthanasia and assisted suicide, what the candidates would do if their own father begged them to help them die, how they would react to a patient asking to help them die and whether it was right to prosecute each case.

5. **A drug company who had been found to organise testing on live animals in a far-flung country not affected by anti-vivisection legislation.**

    The discussions consisted of exploring the issue of vivisection, possible alternatives, whether research would be seriously affected by anti-vivisection legislation and whether all animals could be considered on an equal level to humans.

Essentially, discussions around newspaper articles are the same as what you might expect in a normal panel interview format, with the exception that you will have had time to prepare your thoughts on the topic. Usually you will get about 7-10 days to read the article and prepare yourself for it. In your preparation, make sure that you consider the issues from all possible angles, i.e. the various protagonists involved but also the impact on society.

Do not simply confine yourself to discussing the ethical side of the situation, but also the feelings of the different people involved.

The best way to prepare for the newspaper article section is to take hot stories from well-known news websites and discuss them with friends and family. You will also need to be very familiar with the fundamental ethical principles (see Section 5.8).

15 Communication role play

15.1 Introduction

The communication role play station consists of a simulated conversation between the candidate and an actor around a given scenario. There are three types of scenarios which tend to be used:

- Counselling someone
- Breaking bad news
- Explaining a concept.

How the role play works

A little time before you get into the room you will be given a brief which will set out some basic information. For example:

A friend has recently told you that he is feeling depressed because he has been experiencing a spell of bad marks at school. You have agreed to talk to him after class.

Or

Your best friend has asked you to be his best man/her bridesmaid, to which you agreed months ago. A week before the wedding, you have been asked by one of your family members, who has been recently diagnosed with cancer, to accompany him to hospital, a request which you cannot refuse. You need to tell your friend.

Or

A 9-year-old child tells you that they have heard someone talk about human genes and asks you what this means. Explain it to them.

Opposite you in the room will be either a professional actor or a member of the panel playing the role of the person you are supposed to be talking to. They will also have received their own brief and will behave according to that brief.

So for example, in the case of the 9-year child asking about human genes, the actor may be playing a particularly bright child asking too many questions, or on the contrary a very puzzled child who keeps telling you that he doesn't understand what you are saying.

Similarly, if you are given a role play where you have to break bad news to someone, then they might react by staying completely silent or, on the other hand, getting very angry.

Generally speaking you will not be told what behaviour you can expect before you get into the room. So you should be prepared to face any situation.

What the communication role play tests

The communication role play aims to test a range of communication skills including your ability to:

- Listen
- Show empathy, i.e. to take in others' perspective and treat others with understanding
- Explain ideas in a way that your audience understands
- Communicate effectively and sensitively with others
- Build rapport
- Support and motivate others
- Recognise your own mistakes and learn from them
- Accept feedback constructively and learn from it
- Deal effectively with criticism.

15.2 The "counselling" role play

In a 'counselling' role play, you will be required to provide advice and /or support to an actor playing the role of a friend or relative who has been affected by a particular event.

Examples

Examples of briefs that have come up in the past include:

- A friend confides in you that they have started taking recreational drugs regularly at weekends. You have noticed that their performance at school is deteriorating. Talk to them.

- Your best friend tells you that they are thinking of dropping out of university. Talk to them.

- Your friend tells you that they have been selling pirated DVDs for the past 2 years and that they are scared because one of their own friends has been arrested recently for the same offence.

- Your friend tells you that they have recently been diagnosed with a terminal form of cancer and, at most, they have 18 months to live. Talk to them.

How to handle the role play

The main premise of the counselling role play is that someone has something to tell you; in fact they almost always have initiated the meeting themselves. Therefore you will need to:

- Make sure that the setting is right. For example, if you are given a desk and two chairs facing each other, you might want to move the chairs so that you are both sitting closer to one another and not facing each other (either get rid of the table, or move the chairs so that they are on adjacent sides of the table).

- Let them talk and express their feelings. Resist the temptation to interrupt and ask questions.

- Show that you are listening by
  - Maintaining good eye contact
  - Nodding in the right places
  - Adopting appropriate facial expressions
  - Resisting the temptation to offer your opinion too readily
  - Not being afraid of silence. Sometimes silence is good and it encourages people to talk more
  - Giving occasional short acknowledgment: "Hmm", "Okay", "I understand".

- Ask open questions if you can. For example: "You said you were worried about xxx. What exactly worries you about telling your family?" or "What happened when you told your parents?" or "How do you feel you can get yourself out of this situation?"

- Avoid offering your own judgement or opinions in a manner which is too direct. For example, instead of saying "I think it might be a good idea for you to go and see your GP about this", you could phrase it as "Have you considered seeking help, for example from your GP?"

- When dealing with emotional situations, consider the following four factors: physical, financial, social and psychological. Not all of them are always relevant to every situation but this is a useful checklist to remember to address the different facets. Examples of questions include:

Physical
- How painful is it?
- How are you sleeping?
- Are you experiencing any nasty side effects?

Financial
- How are you managing to pay for 8 pints of beer per night (or x grams of cocaine a week)?
- How does that affect your Saturday job and your income-earning ability?
- Can you afford to take so much time off?

Social
- Who is at home with you?
- Is there anyone you can talk to on a regular basis?
- How is this impacting on your relationship?

Psychological
- Is there anything which is stressing you?
- How are you coping?
- How is this affecting you?

- Test the other person's expectations. For example, they may simply want to vent (in which case you merely sit there and listen, and encourage them to talk by asking suitable open questions), or they may want something more, e.g. for you to take some kind of action to help them. Asking questions such as "Is there anything you would like me to do for you?" can be helpful without committing yourself or imposing your help onto them.

- Think about possible hidden agendas. For example, a friend who is suggesting that they wish to drop out of university may wish to do so for different reasons. Perhaps they have difficulty coping with a life event, or are being bullied.

- Try to finish the conversation on a positive note. This could be, for example, by arranging another meeting later on to discuss how they are doing: "Why don't you see how things go and perhaps we can talk again later on this week." Or by trying to define some kind of action plan (but again through asking questions rather than imposing your point of view). For example: "So, in view of everything we have talked about, what do you feel is your best way forward?" or "How do you plan to handle it with your parents?"

Dealing with an angry person

It may be that the role play leads to the other person turning against you (for example, if the situation is that of a customer in a shop who has come in to complain). If you are starting to feel irritated, if the actor becomes angry or is not listening to you, do not be tempted to show your true feelings. Your emotions will be detectable to the actor and to the interviewers. Recognise them early and take a deep breath. Pause and give yourself time to calm down. A good way of getting out of a sticky situation is to reflect the emotion back to the person that you are with.

- I see you are really angry about this.
- I'm sorry you feel so annoyed about this.
- What can I do to stop you feeling so angry about this?

Such comments will hopefully encourage the actor to talk for a little longer, giving you even more time to compose yourself, calm down and think of another approach. Try it, practise and work out which phrases work for you. Use your own words. Make it part of your everyday conversational style.

Dealing with an emotional person

If the actor starts crying, give them time. Stay silent for a little while (say 20 seconds) and resist the temptation to fill the space. If there are tissues available, offer them one. If there aren't, pretend there are some and hand them an imaginary tissue. Your efforts will be appreciated.

15.3 The "breaking bad news" role play

In a 'breaking bad news' role play. the candidate needs to tell an actor that something bad has happened. There are two parts to this type of role play: breaking the news and dealing with the consequences.

Examples include:

- You have just run over your neighbour's cat whilst reversing your car. You have just rung her bell and she has now opened the door. Talk to her.

- Your best friend asked you to bake her wedding cake. On the morning of the wedding, you proudly present the cake to your friend who asks you whether you had remembered that she has coeliac disease, i.e. the cake needed to be gluten free. You had forgotten all about it. Talk to her.

- You had agreed to go on holiday with your best friend, touring a far-flung country. As you are about to set off, you re-read your travel documents thoroughly and realise that you need a visa to enter the country you wanted to visit. You had not thought about it before and it is now too late to get a visa as it takes at least 3 weeks to obtain one. Talk to your friend.

- You need to tell your family that you really want to be a doctor. Your mother is totally against it. Talk to her.

Breaking the news

- Make sure the setting is right, when breaking bad news; for example, telling an elderly person that you have just run over their cat might be better done when they are sitting down than standing up in the door frame. So if the role play starts at the door, you may want to get in quickly with a sentence of the type "Good morning Mrs X. I wanted to have a quick word with you about something important. Do you mind if I come in?"

- Be honest about the situation. Go for the truth instead of the white lie. For example, don't be tempted to say:

363

> I am not sure how it happened Mrs X, but I found your cat in the street. It looks like he has been run over by some unscrupulous driver.

I know it might be tempting and might seem harmless but integrity and honesty are very important attributes of a doctor and you will not be forgiven for lying, even if it may seem that you can get away with it. You may actually be shown the door before you complete the role play. Instead you might consider something such as:

> I wanted to tell you that I made a mistake whilst reversing my car and that, unfortunately, it seems that your cat Percy was in the path of the car. I tried everything I could but I was unable to revive him and he hasn't made it. I am terribly sorry about it and I feel really bad about it.

- Don't try to invent some very convoluted stories to explain the unexplainable or worse, which blame the wrong person for it. Examples of these would be "Unfortunately the cat jumped right under my wheels" or "That only happened because the cat was let loose and wasn't looking."

- Give the person time to take in the news. Emphasise how sorry you are and how bad you feel about how you have let them down. Whatever you do, position your answers from their perspective and their feelings. For example:

> - I feel that I have really let you down
> - Is there anything that I can do to make it up to you?
> - I would like to make it up to you
> - I can understand that you are angry with me. Once again I can't say enough how sorry I am.

- If there is a possibility of making it up easily to the person, then offer to do so. For example, the friend who has lost money because you messed up with the visas would appreciate a reimbursement of his money. The friend whose cake you didn't do with gluten-free flour may appreciate an offer to bake a new cake just for her quickly – there may still be time and if she is the only one who needs a gluten-free diet, you only need to make a small one especially for her. The other guests can eat the normal cake. It wouldn't be the same but it would be a good compromise.

15.4   The "explaining a concept" role play

In an 'explaining a concept' role play, the candidate is required to explain a concept, or describe an object to an actor, who can play the role of an individual of all ages. Examples include:

- Explain to a 5-year-old child how to tie shoe laces (or how to wrap a parcel). You are not allowed to use your hands.

- Describe this room to a blind person.

- Describe this picture to me:

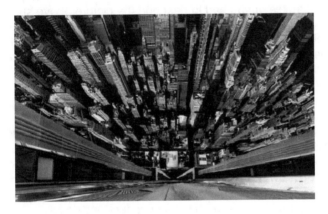

- Describe this diagram to me:

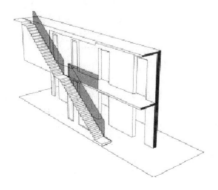

How to handle the role play

This type of role play is meant to test your ability to explain seemingly complex issues in a manner that can be understood by your audience. In doing so, you must pay attention to the following:

- Check who the audience is. You don't explain something to a 5-year-old in the way you explain it to an adult. Similarly, if you are asked to explain something to an adult, you may provide different explanations to someone who has a given amount of prior knowledge than to someone who hasn't.

- Break down your explanations into simple clear steps. See if you can make some analogies with objects or places that the other person knows. For example, if you had to describe the picture above showing the tall buildings to an adult, you could start your explanations by "Imagine being in New York flying over the town in a helicopter". If you had to explain it to a small child, you might assume they are more familiar with Japanese cartoons than helicopter flights over New York and explain the sense of perspective by talking about rays of light coming out of weapons and aiming for a single point in the distance.

- Check that the person understands what you are saying. It would be awful to realise after 5 minutes that they lost the plot 4 minutes previously. To do that, look at their body language, look at their eye contact and their level of awareness, and ask occasionally if they have understood you so far. If you are explaining a practical task, you could even ask them to repeat to you what they have understood so far.

- Occasionally stop and ask if the person has any questions so far or if there are parts of the explanation that they would like to hear again. If the actor or interviewer frowns, show that you are attentive by asking something of the type "I can see that you are frowning. Is there anything which you would like me to explain again?"

- If someone really does not get a point that you have made, you might want to consider explaining it in a different way. In particular, in some cases it may be possible to switch to a different analogy or to switch to a different medium. Check in particular if there is any spare paper lying around; that might be a clue that you could use it to draw a diagram (which is particularly useful if you have to explain something that is technical or scientific).

16 Critique of a video doctor-patient consultation

In some MMI interviews, candidates are shown a short video of a medical consultation – usually a GP addressing a patient or a specialist doctor breaking bad news to a patient – and are asked to comment on the consultation.

These videos are nearly always addressing the same issues, i.e. a doctor who is demonstrating both some very good behaviours and some very bad behaviours. In that station, all you need to do is point out what was done well and what could have been handled differently.

Here is a checklist of points that you need to consider:

1. Is the environment suitable for the consultation?

- Are the doctor and the patient positioned properly, i.e. not facing each other with a table in between, but at a 90° angle as follows?

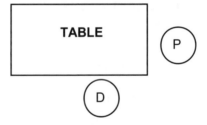

- If there is no table, a similar principle applies. Are the chairs facing each other (bad) or at an angle (better)?

- Is the doctor talking to the patient in a public space (e.g. reception or a corridor within earshot of other patients), risking a breach of privacy and confidentiality?

- Has the doctor switched off his phone and made sure he isn't interrupted? You won't necessarily see that he has done it, but look out for mobile phones ringing in the middle of the consultation, and people interrupting the consultation by storming into the room inappropriately. That would be important for all consultations out of respect for the patient, but of the utmost importance when breaking bad news.

2. Introduction and building a rapport
- Has the doctor introduced himself/herself?
- Is the doctor using the patient's name (e.g. "Hello Mrs X")?
- Has the doctor shaken the patient's hand and asked them nicely to take a seat?
- Generally speaking, is the doctor treating the patient with respect?

3. Active listening
- Is the doctor talking at the patient rather than allowing the patient to talk? Does he understand that silence is sometimes better than words (this is particularly relevant in the more emotional consultations)?
- Is the doctor using open questions or directing the conversation? (You are looking for phrases such as "How can I help you today?")
- Is the doctor visibly listening to the patient? Look for nodding, eye contact, general open body language, interested look on the doctor's face, etc. With the arrival of computers in every consulting room, one common mistake many doctors do is to look at their screen and type whilst the patient talks, meaning they have barely any eye contact.
- Is the doctor encouraging the patient to expand by reflecting on their own words? Look for phrases of the type "You said you were worried about...", "Tell me more about ..." or "What happened afterwards?"
- Is the doctor rushing the patient because he is running late? In some cases, it may be appropriate to redirect the patient (particularly if he is rambling on and giving too much or irrelevant detail) but this needs to be done in a tactful manner.

4. Psychosocial aspect
- Is the doctor just focusing on the obvious or is he interested in elucidating relevant psychosocial information? So for example, if a patient tells the doctor that they would like some sleeping pills because they find it hard to sleep, is the doctor simply prescribing the sleeping pills or is he enquiring about whether they are stressed, are going through a tough time at work or socially, or whether anything has changed in their life recently which may explain why they are finding it hard to sleep? (Basically, is the doctor

interested in the patient as a whole and not just dealing with the symptoms?)

5. Patient's expectations and hidden agenda

- Is the doctor involving the patient and asking what their expectations are? For example, a patient with sleeping problems may not actually want to take medication for it.
- Does it look like the patient has a hidden agenda that the doctor is missing (usually because he is not listening or not asking questions which are open enough)? For example, a patient who seems to have only just come to have a broad chat about their health may actually be lonely and depressed.

6. Explanations and plan of action

- Is the doctor explaining things in a way that the patient understands? Watch the patient's body language when the doctor is explaining and look out for any jargon the doctor might be using.
- Is the doctor checking that the patient has understood what was said? Look out for phrases such as "Do you know what I mean by 'viral infection'?" or "What do you understand when I use the word 'cancer'?" or "Is there anything that you would like me to explain again or in a different way?"
- Is the doctor giving the patient the opportunity to ask questions? Is he answering those questions in a manner that indicates he actually cares?
- Does the consultation conclude with a clear idea of what will happen next?

7. Interaction with others

In some cases, there may be other people present in the consultation room, such as nurses or medical students. If that is the case, look out for the following:

- Is the doctor polite towards those present (e.g. nurses) or is he patronising and/or rude?
- If there are medical students in the room, is he just ignoring them or is he using the consultation to teach them?
- Has the doctor checked with the patient that they are happy to have those extra people in the room during the consultation?

369

17 Group discussion

Regardless of their format, the aim of a group discussion is to test your communication, team playing and leadership skills, and particularly your ability to:

- Present intelligent and informed arguments in a structured and convincing manner.
- Listen to other participants and ensure balance within the group.
- Respect other people's views and play to their strengths.
- Handle differences of opinion constructively.
- Lead the discussion to a practical conclusion, preferably through consensus.
- Handle different personalities successfully, including both passive and active extremes.
- Be mindful of group dynamics.

To perform well, you will therefore need to have thought about current issues and their impact on your specialty, with a particular focus on practical solutions (though one would assume you would have done so already as part of your preparation for the panel interview anyway).

During the discussion, you will need to ensure that you remain open-minded whilst still showing confidence in the way in which you present your own opinions; you will need to make sure also that you listen attentively and respect other people's opinions.

It is perfectly acceptable for you to take the lead (particularly if no one else rises to the challenge) but, in doing so, make sure that you do not take the group over and present yourself as being too overbearing.

Here is an example of a marking structure which is often used to score group discussions:

Competency	Criteria	Mark (out of 5)
Participation	▪ Participates enthusiastically in discussion.	
Spoken Expression	▪ Expresses him/herself clearly and coherently.	
Originality of Ideas	▪ Introduces new ideas. ▪ Builds constructively on the ideas of others. ▪ Brings a fresh approach to a problem.	
Quality of Thought	▪ Analyses the problem well. ▪ Gets to the root of the problem.	
Influence on Others	▪ Makes a point which is accepted. ▪ Influences the direction and nature of the discussion.	
Open-Mindedness	▪ Listens carefully to other members' views. ▪ Incorporates the points made by others into their own.	
Facilitation of the Discussion	▪ Makes a direct attempt to help another person. ▪ Squashes a dominant interrupter to allow someone else to make a point.	
Judgement	▪ Discriminates clearly between the important and the trivial. ▪ Does not allow his/her feelings to sway decisions.	

The roles different people play in meetings and discussions

People may assume different roles in meetings, the most common of which are listed below. These roles are not always constant – one person might adopt several of these roles during one meeting or change roles depending on what is being discussed. Use the descriptions below to determine which roles would best suit your personality:

1. **Encouragers**

   They energise groups when motivation is low through humour or being enthusiastic. They are positive individuals who support and praise other group members. They don't like sitting around. They like to move things along by suggesting ideas, clarifying the ideas of others and confronting problems. They may use humour to break tensions in the group. They may say:

   - "We CAN do this!"
   - "That's a great idea!"

2. **Compromisers**

   They try to maintain harmony among the team members. They are sociable, interested in others and will introduce people, draw them out and make them feel comfortable. They may be willing to change their own views to get a group decision. They work well with different people and can be depended on to promote a positive atmosphere, helping the team to gel. They pull people and tasks together, developing rapport. They are tolerant individuals and good listeners who will listen carefully to the views of other group members. They are good judges of people, diplomatic and sensitive to the feelings of others and not seen as a threat. Able to recognise and resolve differences of opinion and the development of conflict, they enable "difficult" team members to contribute positively. They may say:

   - "We haven't heard from Mike yet: I'd like to hear what you think about this."
   - "I'm not sure I agree. What are your reasons for saying that?"

3. **Leaders**

   Good leaders direct the sequence of steps the group take and keeps the group "on-track". They are good at controlling people and events and coordinating resources. They have the energy, determination and initiative to overcome obstacles and bring competitive drive to the team. They give shape to the team effort. They recognise the skills of the individuals and how they can be used. Leaders are outgoing individuals who have to be careful not to be domineering. They can sometimes steamroller the team but get results quickly. They may become impatient with complacency and lack of progress and may sometimes overreact. They may say:

- "Let's come back to this later if we have time."
- "John, what do you think about this idea?"

4. Summarisers/Clarifiers
They are calm, reflective individuals who summarise the group's discussions and conclusions. They clarify group objectives and elaborate on the ideas of others. They may go into detail about how the group's plans would work and tie up loose ends. They are good mediators and seek consensus. They may say:

- "So here's what we've decided so far"
- "I think you're right, but we could also add ...."

5. Ideas Generators
The ideas person suggests new ideas to solve group problems or new ways for the group to organise the task. They dislike orthodoxy and are not too concerned with practicalities. They provide suggestions and proposals that are often original and radical. They are more concerned with the big picture than with details. They may get bored after the initial impetus wears off. They may say:

- "Why don't we consider doing it this way?"

6. Evaluators
Evaluators help the group avoid coming to agreement too quickly. They tend to be slow in coming to a decision because of the need to think things over. They are the logical, analytical, objective people in the team and offer measured and dispassionate critical analysis. They contribute at times of crucial decision making because they are capable of evaluating competing proposals. They may suggest alternative ideas. They may say:

- "What other possibilities are there?"
- "Let's try to look at this in another way."
- "I'm not sure we're on the right track."

7. Recorders

The recorder keeps the group focused and organised. They make sure that everyone is helping with the project. They are usually the first person to offer to take notes to keep a record of ideas and decisions. They also like to act as time-keeper, to allocate times to specific tasks and remind the team to keep to them, or as spokesperson, to deliver the ideas and findings of the group. They may check that all members understand and agree on plans and actions and know their roles and responsibilities. They act as the memory of the group. They may say:

- "We only have 5 minutes left; we need to conclude soon!"
- "Do we all understand this chart?"
- "Are we all in agreement on this?"

Handling the group discussion

The discussion itself may go in different directions depending on the members present in the group and their personalities; as such, no firm preparation is required. Simply make sure that you are able to put your arguments across in a sensible and organised manner and that you do not take over the group. It is a matter of balance. You may find it beneficial to think about how you may handle different scenarios as and when they develop so that you do not get caught off guard. Here are a few situations that you may wish to think about:

1. The quiet participant

You: You will be assessed on your contribution and participation to the discussion. Melting into the background is not an option. If you are normally quiet and reserved, make an effort to participate. You don't need to be the leader but you need to contribute intelligently. If you are really struggling to get into the debate, start by acknowledging a particular point made by a colleague and build on it. For example: "I totally agree with what you say. I wondered if we could also consider ..."

Another individual: If a member of the group is quiet, see if you can take some action to involve them. There are several reasons why someone may not participate, including the following:

- They are worried they might say something silly.
- They don't have any ideas.
- They have not been listening.

- They can't seem to find the right opportunity to come into the discussion.
- They are just shy and content with listening.
- They are reflectors and may need time to forge an opinion based on the discussion.
- They are deliberately playing a quiet role to see how you react.

In all cases, you will be rewarded for making an effort to involve that colleague in the discussion. They may decline your invitation but at least you will have tried. If you do decide to involve a quiet colleague into the discussion, try to do so in a way that does not embarrass them. Phrases such as "You seem to be quiet; what do you think about this topic" may seem a little overwhelming to someone who is content with taking a back seat. Equally, asking someone to summarise the situation when they have in fact not been listening will send them into a panic. You don't want to be perceived as someone who has no problem embarrassing a colleague.

Instead, try to ask their opinion on a narrow part of the topic, which relates to an area with which they are familiar and may not necessarily require a good understanding of prior discussions. So for example, saying "Do you have any opinion?" may feel threatening. But asking "Sarah thinks that PBL is a good idea because it promotes teamwork whereas John thinks it can't work unless it is combined with formal lectures. What would be your inkling?"

2. **The loud participant**
   You: If you are the type of individual who tends to talk a lot or who always takes the lead, take a step back and think about the situation. You may think that you have all the good ideas but this task is about a lot more than appearing intelligent and creative. It is also testing your interaction with the whole group. Are you listening to the others? Is there someone else who looks like they would like to take over for a while? Try offering the lead to other people. Look at the other participants and their body language. If everyone is included and happy, it will be evident from their behaviour and body language. If people are looking away, are disengaging or, worse, start talking amongst themselves, then something is going wrong. If you feel that you may be coming across as overbearing, see if you can find a way of passing the baton on to someone else. Phrases such as "I apologise if I seem to have taken rather a long time to put my thoughts across; would someone else like to comment and give us their perspective on the issue?"

Another individual: If you face a situation where one member of the group is taking over, making others feel uncomfortable, there are ways to ease the awkwardness that it creates:

- Try opening the floor to others: "Asim, I am not sure that I agree with you on every point. My opinion would be that <give opinion>. What do you think, Sarah?" By doing so, you are bringing another voice into the conversation. This often reminds dominant colleagues that there are other people around.
- Try changing the subject: "We are halfway through our time for the meeting. Does anyone mind if I summarise where we are up to?"
- If the loud colleague simply does not get the message or is unstoppable, you may need to be a little more direct: "Paula, I think that you have very good arguments and certainly I am inclined to agree with you on the fact that <mention what you are agreeing with>. But it might be a good idea if we went round the table and obtained everyone else's point of view as there may be aspects of the question that we may have missed." By mentioning that you are partially agreeing with them, you will soothe the tension a little and what comes next will not appear to be so threatening to the individual in question. If you don't agree with anything they have mentioned, you can say: "There is quite a lot to take in amongst what you said, and it may be an idea to deal with one issue at a time. Perhaps we could go round the table and see if anyone would like to add to what has just been mentioned."

3. Conflict

It is most unlikely that you will agree with everything that is being said during the group discussion and it is perfectly acceptable to disagree with your colleagues provided you can substantiate your own opinion. Don't try to fight a battle on a matter of principle; it won't appear very clever. If you do not agree, say so, but do it in a way that shows that you respect and value your colleague's contribution: "This is an interesting point, but I am not sure that it can necessarily be generalised"; "I am not sure I am entirely comfortable with this concept."

You: If you find yourself being the one who is causing a conflict or says something out of turn, back down graciously. Think about the good functioning of the team rather than your pride: "I am sorry. I was getting a little overexcited then"; "I think I need to step back. What do you think about this issue George?"

Another individual: If another candidate is being offensive or deliberately obtrusive, see if you can diffuse the situation: "I am not sure if we will find a solution with this approach; shall we move on to <change the subject> and perhaps we can get back to this issue later?"; "You both seem very passionate about this issue. I am not sure we can reach a conclusion without more thoughts on the topic. Shall we talk about xxx?"

4. Recurrent themes – going round in circles

If you find that the group is constantly going over the same ground or has gone way off topic, try to bring the focus of the discussion back to the brief: "This is really interesting but I am not sure this is strictly related to the topic that we are trying to address"; "Sorry; I think I am a bit lost. Can we recap?"

5. Trouble finishing the discussion

However tempting it may be to assume that there is a consensus about the topic and future action needed, think carefully about how you wish to conclude the discussions as this will drastically influence the manner in which you are perceived. Last impressions count. Phrases that would contribute to a positive image include:

- "I think we have covered everything. Is everyone happy with the approach that we have discussed?"
- "Does anyone have anything else to add? Shall we draw the meeting to a close? Does everyone agree?"

During the meeting you should keep a careful eye on the clock (if there is no clock, then place your watch on the table discreetly so that you can glance at it occasionally without having to look at your wrist). If you see that you are running short of time, try to encourage the group to move on: "We seem to have only 5 minutes left. Shall we move on to the next issue?" As you approach the end of the allotted time, make sure that the group draws up some kind of action plan. This might include real work to be carried out by some members of the team or simply to agree to hold a follow-up meeting to discuss any outstanding issues. If you feel that some issues do not need to be discussed by the whole group and could be more productively discussed by a subgroup instead, suggest that people meet separately and then report to the whole group later on. This will make you appear efficient.

18 Group task

Group or team exercises involve working physically with other candidates to the post to resolve a particular issue, ranging from discussing a practical matter to undertaking a physical task together.

Exercises used by some medical schools in the recent past have included:

Building a robot or rocket using a set of Lego blocks
Candidates are split into two groups. One group has the instructions but not the building blocks; the other group has the building blocks but not the instructions. Both teams need to work together to complete the task.

Building an object
Given 4 plastic cups, 4 plates, masking tape and 8 sheets of very large paper, construct a bridge capable of holding a stapler (the stapler isn't seen until you've finished).

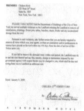

Handling a complaint
Candidates are given a complaint letter together with a set of patient notes. They need to discuss the situation and establish a way forward to ensure a positive outcome. In some cases, candidates may be required to complete this task individually (i.e. every candidate must produce a response letter to the complaint).

Such exercises are still relatively uncommon, mainly because they require a lot of well-trained observers to make any sense of the outcome. They assess similar skills to group discussions and, as such, you should follow the same rules (see Section 17).

19 Prioritisation exercise

Usually, prioritisation exercises involve giving candidates a situation and a challenge, which requires making hard choices. In general the questions are rarely difficult if you demonstrate some common sense and remember that, should you need more information, you can always ask the interviewers.

Here are a few examples and ideas on how to handle them:

1. **You are given a list of the 30 items contained in your suitcase. At the airport check-in you are being told that your suitcase is over the weight limit and that you need to offload 15 of the 30 items. How would you go about deciding which ones you keep?**

    The first thing you will need to do is scan the list of items and ask the interviewers where you are supposed to be going as this will inevitably weed out a number of obviously unsuitable items. For example, you will not need to take mosquito-repellent cream if you are travelling to Iceland in the winter.

    Next you will need to consider how easily you will be able to purchase some of the items once you have reached your destination. For example, there is no point packing shaving foam and toothpaste if you buy it on arrival, especially if that means that you can no longer take other items which may be more expensive (such as a coat).

    Then think about what constitutes an essential item and a luxury. For example, you might not need 3 pairs of trousers if you are going away for just 5 days, unless you are going on an adventure holiday where you may get soaked easily. The same goes for shoes.

    For example, if you are going to a place where you can buy basic items once you have reached your destination then you may not need to take those basics with you. Think also about which items would be essential but may not be available on site.

379

2. **You are given a list of 15 individuals including their gender, age and occupation. You can save 5 of them from a nuclear attack. How would you go about deciding which ones you save?**

In your answer consider the following factors:

- If there are only 5 people left, you will need them to be healthy. Choosing people who have a short life expectancy may cause problems for the survival of the group.

- You need a mix of experienced people (i.e. middle-aged) and also younger ones (to reproduce and ensure continuity of the race). For the latter you will also need mixed genders.

- You need to choose people from a variety of trades. At this stage, people with manual skills are probably more useful than those with administrative skills (5 people don't require an administrator to survive!). That would include anyone with knowledge of carpentry (or building work generally), agriculture/gardening, fishing and possibly medicine.

3. **You are travelling on the London underground with a group of 5 other people. One of the members of the group becomes separated from the others. They have no mobile phone on them, have no map on them and have never been to London before. Describe your plan of action.**

- There are two possibilities: either your friend finds his own way back to the hotel or he can't. If he does then it may be a good idea for someone to be there waiting for them and ready to let the others know that he has been found.

- It is likely that you will need to split up in order to find your friend (there is little value in staying together); however, you should all attempt to stay in contact with each other, either by phone if you have them, or by agreeing a meeting place and a meeting time to compare notes.

- One person could go to the station master so that they can make an announcement, and also possibly inform the police (they might look out for them).

- One person could retrace the steps taken by the group to see if the friend can be found. It is always possible that the friend remained static or at least did not stray far from a previously visited destination.

- Ultimately there is little you can do if your friend is really lost other than hope they will remember where the hotel is and that they will ask someone for directions but in your answer you must demonstrate that you are able to come up with some ideas that may yield immediate results (for example, making an announcement quickly would be ideal so that your friend hears it before they move on).

These questions do not often have a single answer. The interviewers will be more interested in your thought process than in the actual answer, so make sure that you explain why you have made your choices.

20 Data analysis exercise

In this task, candidates are given a paper to read before entering the interview room. The paper usually contains information displayed in the form of tables or graphs, but may also contain wordy information. Candidates are asked to answer questions requiring them to draw conclusions from the data given.

Here are a few examples of graphs, which were given to candidates in recent years:

Example 1

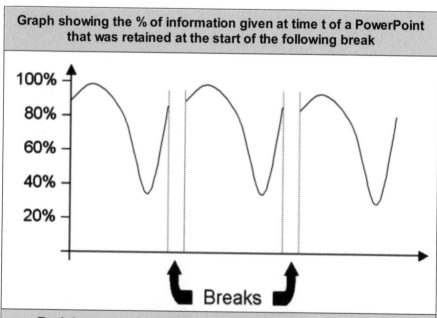

Graph showing the % of information given at time t of a PowerPoint that was retained at the start of the following break

Each interval lasts 50 minutes, each break lasts 10 minutes.
What can you conclude from this graph?

Suggested answer:

1. The graph shows that the information most people remember is that given approximately 10 minutes after the start of the presentation. Since it happens in a cyclical way, i.e. we observe the same pattern after each break, this suggests that the break has a positive impact on information retention.

2. Attention span seems to pick up 10 minutes before the break. This would suggest either that people have a natural tendency to "wake up" after 40 minutes (maybe because they are trying to wake themselves up), or more likely that they know that a break is coming up and therefore they suddenly start to wake up. It is also possible that the final 10 minutes of a presentation before a break consists of some kind of summary, and therefore might sound more interesting than the bulk of the presentation itself.

3. *Follow up question from the interviewers:* How would that graph help you improve your own presentations?

   Answer: This suggests that there should be frequent breaks and that a gap of 30 minutes between breaks would help maintain attention at high levels throughout the presentation (though there is a risk it then become bitty and people start losing patience with it).

4. *Follow up question from the interviewers:* Can we conclude from this graph that breaks should be no more than 10 minutes?

   Answer: After a break, the line of attention span is the same as it was at the very start of the presentation. This suggests that a 10-minute break resets you to the same attention level as you were at the very start. However, without having a similar graph for breaks of say 5 and 15 minutes, we cannot come to a definitive conclusion.

Example 2

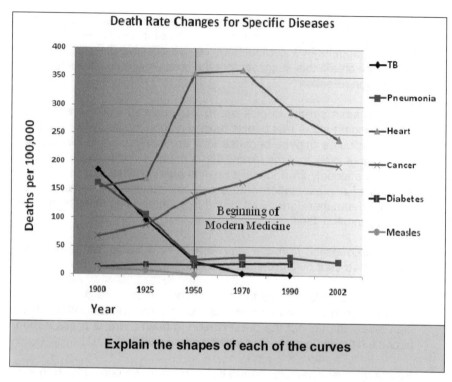

Death Rate Changes for Specific Diseases

Beginning of Modern Medicine

Explain the shapes of each of the curves

Suggested answer:

1. The curve for heart disease is clearly on the up before the beginning of modern medicine, it plateaus for about 20 years until 1970 and then it is on a sharp downwards trend thereafter. The trend upwards is most likely linked to bad diet and lifestyle habits, and the trend downwards to the introduction of suitable medication and surgery. In the early 1970s there seems to have been a key discovery, which changed the course of heart disease. (Note: statin drugs which help control cholesterol were actually introduced in 1971.)

2. Deaths from cancer went up throughout the period and then slightly decrease after 1990. This is likely due to the fact that the population is getting older and therefore more prone to cancer; basically as fewer people die of other diseases (such as heart disease) they are dying of

cancer instead. The slight tail off in the 1990s corresponds most likely to the introduction of better cancer treatments.

3. Deaths from tuberculosis (TB) have been on a steady decline since well before the onset of modern medicine. This suggests that this was due to an earlier vaccine (in fact the vaccine for TB was first used in 1921) and possibly also to improved living conditions due to modernisation. Deaths from pneumonia have also fallen steadily throughout the entire period, most likely due to improvement in living conditions.

4. Death from diabetes remained very low and stable throughout the whole period, though with a slightly upward trend. This suggests it has been controlled from an early stage (in fact insulin was introduced in the 1920s).The slight increase may come from the fact that, though diabetes is better controlled now, this has likely been counteracted by an increase in cases due to a worsening of eating habits. It is also possible that there is a link between the heart disease curve and the diabetes curve since it may affect the same people. So as the heart disease curve drops, it may make the diabetes curve rise.

5. The drop in the rate of deaths due to measles suggests that this may be due to the introduction of a new vaccine. However, this does not make sense as the measles vaccine was only introduced in 1968 in the UK. In reality the reasons for this decrease before the introduction of the vaccine are still being debated somewhat but it is believed that the survival from measles was higher due to better nutrition and living conditions.

Important note: you can see that the answer above contains a number of facts which you may or may not know. It is not important that you should know them but a little bit of general medical culture can't hurt. More importantly, what matters is that you are able to brainstorm and find ideas. The interviewers can then guide you along. For example, on the issue of measles, most people would have concluded that a vaccine must have become available in the 1950s. That would be a sensible point to make. The interviewers would then point to the fact that this wasn't even the case and may then ask you to guess a possible explanation.

Lateral thinking and common sense should guide you towards a lot of the answers though.

Example 3 (you don't have a calculator)

Q: What kind of vehicle could this be?

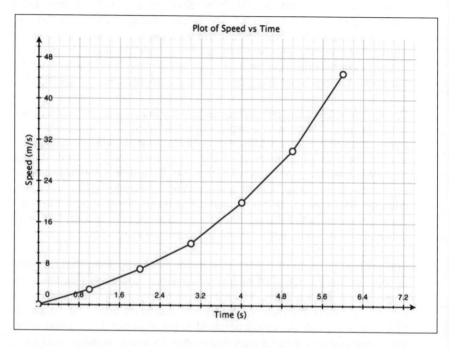

A: The speed reached at 6 seconds is 45 m/s. Let's say 40 to make it easy to calculate. That represents 40 x 60 x 60 = 144,000 m/h, i.e. 144 km/h or roughly 90 miles/h. So that could just be a car.

BODY LANGUAGE

&

DRESS CODE

21 Body language

Much has been written about body language and you may find various statistics quoted, such as body language represents about 60% of your communication.

Whilst there is no doubt that body language is important in helping you make a good impression, one should not forget that, ultimately, your body language is a reflection of your confidence and that confidence is not something that you acquire solely by smiling politely and moving your arms properly. There is a danger that a candidate may concentrate heavily on his/her appearance at the expense of building content and structure into his/her answers.

As you gain more and more confidence through your preparation, your body language will change and will open up naturally. I would therefore recommend that you do not worry about it until you are well advanced in your preparation.

The key rules of body language

If your interview consists of several stations of 5-10 minutes each, you will need to build a rapport and make a good impression quickly. Here are a few key rules that you will need to follow:

Eye contact
This is the most crucial part of your relationship with the interviewers as far as body language is concerned. No one will be interested in listening to someone who is not looking straight at them so make sure that you main-tain good eye contact with whoever is asking you the question. Occasion-ally look at the other person too so that they feel included.

Seat position
If you are sitting behind a table, make sure that you are not too close or too far from the table. If you are too close, you will have difficulty relaxing and also your elbows will be forced to rest on the table. The interviewers would feel that you are invading their space and may be forced to back

away from you. If you are too far from the table, you will either start slouching in your seat, giving the impression that you don't really care, or you will lean forward reaching for the table. Not only will you get lower back pains, but you will also appear very casual. A good distance is about 10 cm from the table so that your arms can rest on the table comfortably with the elbows remaining outside the table and not on it.

Arm positions

Many candidates find it comfortable to have their hands under the table. This gives an impression of timidity and of trying to hide behind the furniture. You need to project an image of quiet confidence and having your hands on the table will help you achieve that.

Hand movements

It is perfectly acceptable to move your hands if it is part of your personality. Don't force yourself if it doesn't come naturally to you though. If you are someone whose hands tend to move naturally, make sure that you contain that movement to the space in front of you and no higher than chest level; otherwise your hand movements will start obstructing your face.

22 Dress code

There are hundreds of ways in which you can make a good impression with your dress code. Here are some general rules that will make a difference in the way in which people perceive you though:

Dress smart
It is an interview and therefore a professional meeting. You will be expected to wear a smart suit and not a jumper. Having said that, you are not going to your own wedding; so don't dress over the top. What matters is that you are comfortable in your clothes and that they are fit for the purpose of a professional meeting. It often helps to mirror the dress code of those interviewing you (generally conservative).

Dress to frame your face
The focal point should be your face; therefore you want to frame your face by wearing darker colours on the outside and lighter colours on the inside. For men, this will mean a shirt of light tone and for women a light-coloured blouse. This should be complemented by a dark-toned suit.

Look neat
If you wear a beard, make sure you trim it. If you wear make-up, don't overdo it. Clip your nails, tidy your hair, and make sure none of it obstructs your face. I know it sounds obvious but you would be surprised.

Avoid distracting features
Continuing on the theme of your face being the focal point, avoid any features or accessories which may draw the eye to the wrong places. In particular: no sequins (they make wonderful disco balls when light reflects off them), no brooches, no ribbons, poppies, or other symbols that are either too big or too bright in colour.

Small items of jewellery may be okay providing they do not steal the limelight away from you and do not draw the attention away from your face.

FULL INDEX

OF

QUESTIONS

&

ISSUES